RESPIRATORY PROBLEMS

RN NURSING ASSESSMENT SERIES

RESPIRATORY PROBLEMS

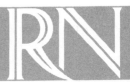

RN NURSING ASSESSMENT SERIES
ELLEN K. BOYDA, R.N., M.S., CCRN

Series Editor
Margaret Van Meter, R.N.
Clinical Editor, RN Magazine

MEDICAL ECONOMICS BOOKS
Oradell, New Jersey 07649

Library of Congress Cataloging in Publication Data

Boyda, Ellen K.
  Respiratory problems.

  (RN nursing assessment series ; 5)
  Bibliography: p.
  Includes index.
  1. Respiratory disease nursing.   I. Title.
II. Series: RN nursing assessment series ; v. 5.
[DNLM: 1. Respiratory Tract Diseases — nursing.
WY 100 R627 1982 v.5]
RC735.5.B69   1985   616.2   84-1187
ISBN 0-87489-282-1

Cover design by Jerry Wilke

ISBN 0-87489-282-1

Medical Economics Company Inc.
Oradell, New Jersey 07649

Printed in the United States of America

CONTENTS

Publisher's Notes — vii

1. Pulmonary Anatomy and Physiology — 1

2. Patient History — 23

3. Respiratory Assessment — 33

4. Arterial Blood Gas Interpretation — 57

5. Chronic Obstructive Pulmonary Disease — 69

6. Restrictive Lung Disease — 83

7. Occupational Lung Diseases — 89

8. Pulmonary Vascular Disease — 103

9. Lung Infections — 113

10. Lung Tumors — 125

11. Chest Trauma — 129

12. Acute Respiratory Failure and Adult Respiratory Distress Syndrome — 137

13. Airway Management — 149

14. Respiratory Therapy Techniques — 165
    Robert J. Boyda, B.S.

15. Mechanical Ventilation — 179

Glossary — 187

Additional Test Questions — 191

Selected Readings — 196

Index — 197

PUBLISHER'S NOTES

Physical assessment is an integral part of the nursing process. Sharpening assessment skills, therefore, is bound to add logic and reason to planning, intervention, and evaluation. This volume in the *RN Nursing Assessment Series* focuses on assessment of respiratory function. In addition to a clear exposition of respiratory physiology, it offers normal parameters against which to compare pathologic findings.

For easy access, an outline format combined with a clear, concise text—an organizational scheme that has proven popular with nurses—was adopted. The illustrations, both halftone and line art, were selected specifically to add to the book's clarity and utility. Finally, the presentation of learning objectives and the inclusion of chapter quizzes, additional test questions, and a glossary make this book a learning/teaching tool.

Ellen K. Boyda, R.N., M.S., CCRN, is an independent clinical specialist in pulmonary nursing and director of pulmonary rehabilitation at Taylor Hospital in Ridley Park, Pennsylvania. She was previously adjunct assistant professor in the Widener University School of Nursing graduate program in Chester, Pennsylvania, and an instructor in critical care at Crozer-Chester Medical Center. With Sally Mowris, R.N., M.S., she earned an *RN* Excellence in Nursing award in 1983 for devising a pulmonary rehabilitation program for patients with chronic obstructive pulmonary disease. Ms. Boyda has also published papers on respiratory assessment and critical care and conducted a number of workshops on these topics. Robert J. Boyda, B.S., the author of Chapter 14, is director of respiratory therapy at Taylor Hospital and for many years has lectured to nurses on respiratory care. Sally Ryan, R.N., who contributed the section on pneumonias in Chapter 9, is nurse epidemiologist at Crozer-Chester Medical Center.

Margaret Van Meter, R.N., the series editor, is RN Magazine's clinical editor for development and also serves as an independent nurse consultant.

1

Pulmonary Anatomy and Physiology

OBJECTIVES

After completing this chapter, you will be able to:

1. *Explain the difference between conducting airways and gas exchange airways*

2. *Explain the principles of negative intrapleural pressure and how it works in the lung*

3. *Describe the role of surfactant in lung function*

4. *List four clinical conditions creating a ventilation-perfusion imbalance*

5. *List the causes of hypoxemia*

6. *Identify the location of central and peripheral chemoreceptors and explain how they work in the neurocontrol of ventilation.*

A. Anatomy

1. Upper airway

All the structures in the upper airway are part of the conducting system through which air moves from the atmosphere into the lungs. The upper airway accounts for about 30 to 50 percent of the anatomic dead space (airways that don't participate in gas exchange) (See Figure 1-1).

a. Nose. The nose has two passageways (nares) separated by the nasal septum. The nose humidifies, heats, and filters the incoming air so that it will not damage the lower airway. The sense of smell is located in the turbinates of the nose.

The narrow nasal passages increase airway resistance, which enables the nose to perform these functions efficiently.

b. Mouth. Although used sometimes for breathing, the mouth is not as effective as the nose because the mouth has a smaller surface area for filtering and does not have ciliated epithelium to help trap the dust and germs from inhaled air.

c. Pharynx (throat). This includes the nasopharynx, above the soft palate; the oropharynx, from the soft palate to the base of the tongue; and the laryngopharynx, below the base of the tongue.

d. Tonsils and adenoids. Located in the back of the throat, they are part of a ring of lymphoid tissue around the throat; they guard against invasion by organisms entering the nose and mouth.

e. Larynx (voice box). The larynx connects the upper airway with the lower airway, protects the lower airway from foreign substances, facilitates coughing, and permits speech — its most important role. It consists of the following:
- Epiglottis — leaf-shaped cartilage that covers the glottis during swallowing
- Glottis — the opening to the trachea
- Thyroid cartilage — "Adam's apple," the largest cartilage in the larynx
- Cricoid cartilage — located below the thyroid cartilage, this is the only complete ring and is the narrowest part

Figure 1-1 *The respiratory system. Reproduced, with permission, from Basics of RD. New York, The American Lung Association, 1980.*

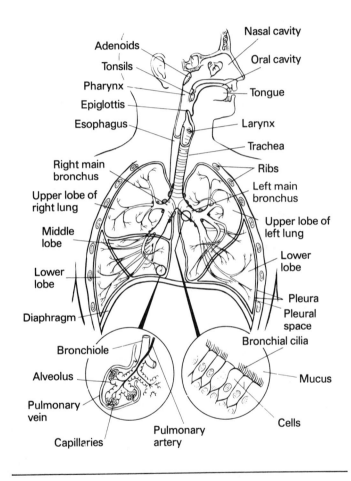

of an infant's or small child's trachea (one reason for cuffless intubation tubes for this age)
• Arytenoid cartilages — used in vocal cord movement with the thyroid cartilage

• Vocal cords — composed of ligamentous and cartilaginous tissue that extends from the arytenoid cartilages to the thyroid cartilage.

2. Tracheobronchial tree

This is the upper part of the lower airway. It consists of three layers:
  • Epithelium — a pseudostratified, ciliated, columnar layer that contains the basement membrane and is lined with many mucous and serous secreting glands
  • Lamina propria (submucosa) — loose, fibrous tissue with small blood and lymphatic vessels and nerves; contains elastic and smooth muscle fibers; this layer contracts, causing increased airway resistance (as in asthma)
  • Cartilaginous layer — varying amounts of cartilage that disappear in airways smaller than 1 mm in diameter (large bronchioles).

The *trachea* (windpipe) lies in front of the esophagus; it measures 11 to 13 cm in length and 1.5 to 2.5 cm in diameter; and it is composed of 16 to 20 C-shaped cartilaginous rings. Since the trachea's posterior wall has no cartilage, you must be careful when inflating a cuff in an intubated patient. Otherwise, the tube could erode the posterior wall, causing a tracheoesophageal fistula.

3. Lower airway

The trachea branches into the right and left mainstem bronchi at the carina, which lies beneath the angle of Louis (where the manubrium joins the sternum, or breastbone).

a. Mainstem bronchi. Histologically these bronchi are similar to the trachea. The *right bronchus* is wider and shorter than the left and branches like an extension of the trachea at a 25-degree angle. This relatively straight line with the trachea makes it easy for an endotracheal tube to enter the right bronchus if it is pushed down too far during intubation. Also, if aspiration occurs, the aspirated substance will most likely enter the right bronchus. However, the straight-line effect makes it easier to enter this bronchus for suctioning purposes.

The *left bronchus* leaves the trachea at a 40- to 60-degree angle. This sharper angle makes accidental intubation as well as suctioning more difficult.

b. Bronchi. There are several divisions:

- Lobar—three on the right and two on the left, making up the lobes of the lung; these tubes are rigid despite absence of C-shaped cartilage
- Segmental—10 on the right and 8 on the left, an important consideration for choosing the most effective postural drainage position for patients
- Subsegmental—generating from the fourth to ninth levels of branching and surrounded by connective tissue that contains arteries, lymphatics, and nerves.

c. Bronchioles. Bronchioles generate from approximately the 9th to 11th levels of branching. These tubes are less than 1 mm in diameter and have no cartilage. Their patency depends entirely upon the elastic recoil of smooth muscle and the level of alveolar pressure.

d. Terminal bronchioles. Terminal bronchioles consist of approximately the 11th to 16th generations of branching and are only 0.5 mm in diameter. They contain no mucous glands or cilia. Any mucus that accumulates here has drained from a higher level in the tracheobronchial tree.

4. Lung parenchyma

The tracheobronchial tree's conducting airways consist of about 150 ml (1 ml/pound of body weight) of anatomic dead space (the volume of inhaled air caught in the tracheobronchial tree that does not participate in gas exchange). The lung parenchyma, the functional respiratory unit, is where the exchange of oxygen and carbon dioxide takes place.

a. Respiratory bronchioles. Forming approximately the 16th to 19th generations of branching, the respiratory bronchioles are viewed as transition passageways between the conducting airways and the gas exchange airways.

b. Alveolar ducts. The alveolar ducts come from the respiratory bronchioles, and half of all the alveoli in the lungs arise directly from these ducts. In alveolar disease, pressure from these alveoli can cause the alveolar ducts to narrow.

c. Primary lobule. Coming directly from the alveolar ducts, this is considered to be the respiratory unit of the lungs. There are approximately 130,000 of these lobules, each 3.5 mm in diameter and containing 2,000 alveoli.

d. Alveolar sacs and alveoli. These are the lung's dead-end passageways. There are about 300 million alveoli occurring in clusters of 15 to 20. Alveoli have common walls, which increase the surface area for gas exchange and also determine the lung's elastic recoil capability. There are three types of alveolar cells: type I (epithelial cells, which form the alveolar wall); type II (metabolically active cells, which are believed to secrete surfactant, a substance that lines the inner surface of the alveoli); and type III (macrophages; these phagocytic cells are part of the lymphatic system).

5. Mucus

The submucosal glands, located in the epithelium of the tracheobronchial tree (goblet cells), produce about 100 ml/day of mucus; this mucus forms an uninterrupted covering for the epithelium of the tracheobronchial tree. Mucus is composed of 95 percent water, 2 percent glycoprotein, 1 percent carbohydrate, and traces of lipids and foreign elements. When irritated, the mucous glands become inflamed and enlarged and secrete more mucus.

The beating action of *cilia* moves mucus up and away from the lower airway. Both cilia and mucus clear the respiratory tract by propelling foreign substances toward the larynx at a rate of 2 cm/minute.

Sputum, which is mobilized by the cough reflex, consists of mucus from the tracheobronchial tree, nasal secretions, and saliva.

6. Alveolar fluid lining

a. Epithelium. The alveolar wall is composed of many alveolar epithelial cells. This epithelium is lined with fluid of unknown origin.

b. Macrophages. These large phagocytic cells, occurring in the alveolar wall, ingest foreign matter (mucus, bacteria) and act as an important defense mechanism.

c. Surfactant. Secreted by cell type II in the alveolar wall, surfactant is a phospholipid, a detergent-like substance that reduces surface tension so the alveoli can remain open and function normally. Surfactant forms a film on the alveolar wall surface and is permeable to all gases. It may be spread, or its production stimulated, by deep inhalation through such techniques as deep breathing, incentive spirometry, and intermittent positive pressure breathing (IPPB). Without surfactant, atelectasis occurs.

7. Thorax

The thorax (chest) contains the lungs, heart, and mediastinal structures such as the great vessels, trachea, esophagus, thymus gland, lymphatics, and nerves.

a. The thoracic cage. Formed by the sternum, ribs, vertebral column, and diaphragm, the thoracic cage houses the structures within the thorax.

b. Lungs. The lungs are encased in the pleural cavity, which lies within the thorax. They are attached to the tracheobronchial tree and emerge from the pleural cavity only at the hilus, where the two mainstem bronchi branch and where the pulmonary vessels enter and leave the thoracic space.

c. Pleura. The pleura has two surfaces. The *parietal pleura*, which lies next to the thoracic cage, has nerve endings that can produce pain when irritated. The *visceral pleura*, which lies next to the lung surface, is without nerve endings and thus is not painful when diseased. These two surfaces oppose each other and are separated by a thin fluid layer which creates negative pressure, thereby causing the lungs to move together with the thoracic cage.

8. Muscles of ventilation

a. Diaphragm. As the major muscle of inspiration, it consists of two muscular hemidomes located at the fifth and sixth rib level anteriorly and at the 10th thoracic vertebra posteriorly. Since the diaphragm is innervated by the phrenic nerve, which branches from the spinal cord at the C_3 to C_5 level, breathing dysfunction must be considered in patients with cervical spine fractures.

b. Intercostal muscles. The internal intercostals play a role in forceful expiration by pulling the ribs down and in; the external intercostals increase the anterior-posterior diameter by elevating the ribs with an outward movement. Both internal and external intercostals are innervated at spinal cord levels T_1 to T_{11}.

c. Abdominal muscles. These muscles are used only during active expiration and coughing (normal expiration is usually passive). They are innervated at spinal cord levels T_6 to L_1.

d. Accessory muscles. This group, which includes the scalene, sternocleidomastoid, trapezius, and pectoralis muscles, is used for breathing only in disease states. These muscles function independently for some inspiration, but they are inefficient because they require more oxygen and a higher level of energy expenditure.

9. Pulmonary and bronchial circulations

a. Pulmonary circulation. This circulation is aligned with the tracheobronchial tree and the alveolar structures almost on a one-to-one basis: For every bronchiole there is a corresponding arteriole and venule, and for every alveolus there is a corresponding capillary. The pulmonary circulation is a low-pressure system (mean pulmonary artery pressure is 10 to 20 mm Hg) and receives the whole cardiac output with each contraction of the heart. It is efficient; each red blood cell spends 4 seconds in the capillary network, where it passes by two or three alveoli and becomes oxygenated before returning through the pulmonary venous circulation to the left of the heart and then to the whole body.

b. Bronchial circulation. This system, which branches off from the aorta, carries the blood supply for the conducting airways (trachea to terminal bronchioles). This circulation enables the lungs to function, but does not participate in gas exchange. The pulmonary and bronchial circulations may be able to anastomose to form collateral circulation whenever needed (as the heart does).

B. Physiology of the lung

1. Ventilation

Ventilation is the act of moving air in and out of the lungs (breathing). The level of ventilation is determined by the lung-thorax relationship, as well as the lung's elastance, compliance, and airway resistance. These factors also affect the volume of air that is in the lung or that exchanges with each breath, the work of breathing, and the distribution of air.

a. Lung-thorax relationship. The natural tendency of the thoracic cage is to be expanded while that of the lung is to be contracted (deflated). The negative intrapleural pressures within the pleural cavity cause the lungs and thoracic cage to work together. On inspiration, the thorax expands, pulling the lung and pleura with it (Figure 1-2). This creates a sucking effect and the pleural pressures become even more negative (relative to atmospheric pressure). At this point the pressure within the lung itself also becomes negative. A pressure gradient is thus created with the air outside the lungs, causing air to fill the lungs as it moves from an area of greater pressure (atmospheric air at sea level is 760 mm Hg) to an area of lesser pressure (approximately 757 mm Hg within the lung tissue). Thus, air fills the lungs until the pressure there is greater than that of the air outside.

Expiration is passive as air moves from an area of greater pressure in the lung to the outside. At the end of expiration, pressure in the lung equals atmospheric pressure; it remains that way until the next inspiration, when the cycle begins again. Lung expansion, therefore, depends on an intact pleural cavity where negative pressure is maintained.

b. Elastance. This is the ability of the lung to recoil or return to its resting state after having been distended. Two of

Figure 1-2 *Intrapleural pressures. Reproduced, with permission, from Harper R: A Guide to Respiratory Care, Philadelphia: Lippincott, 1981.*

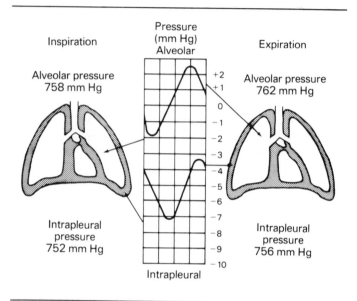

the primary forces that determine the lung's elastance are the interstitial elastic fibers and the fluid that lines the alveolar surface. Since elastic forces work mainly during expiration, there is a tendency for the alveoli to collapse and remain closed. This would lead to massive atelectasis if it were not for surfactant (see section A6 above).

c. Compliance. The opposite of elastance, compliance is the lung's ability to stretch or expand when a force is applied; it allows inspiration to take place. Compliance is determined by the amount of pressure required to deliver a specified volume of air to the lung. A compliant lung requires little pressure to expand easily. A noncompliant lung expands only with great effort as in pulmonary edema, abdominal distention, and fibrosis of the lung.

d. Airway resistance. This determines the rate at which a volume of gas travels in the airways. Generally, the smaller the airway, the greater the resistance to airflow. Airway resistance is increased by constriction or obstruction (e.g., asthma).

e. Lung volumes. Since volumes of air in the lung can be measured (see Figure 1-3), we can evaluate lung function (ventilation). Several of the measurements include:

- Forced vital capacity (FVC) — the same as vital capacity (VC) except that it is achieved by forceful expiration; from it are derived the forced expiratory volume occurring in 1 second (FEV_1), 2 seconds (FEV_2), etc., and the maximum midexpiratory flow rate (MMEFR) — a measure of airway resistance (normal FEV_1 should be about 80 percent of VC)
- Maximum voluntary ventilation (MVV) — the volume of air exhaled per minute with the patient breathing as fast and as deeply as he can
- Minute ventilation (V_E) — the volume of air exhaled in 1 minute (tidal volume times rate)
- Flow-volume curves — a single breath test that measures most of the above volumes; it tends to be more accurate than the traditional volume-time curves of pulmonary function studies (see Table 1-1).

f. Work of breathing. Breathing requires the muscles of ventilation to expend energy. Four clinical factors will increase the work of breathing: decreased compliance (as in pulmonary edema), increased airway resistance (as in asthma), increased active expiration (as in chronic obstructive pulmonary disease), and dramatic change in ventilatory pattern.

g. Distribution of ventilation. In healthy lungs, ventilation is greatest in the lower regions and decreases as you move upward. Besides the regional inequality of ventilation, there is uneven ventilation among alveoli. This is offset in part by little pores (pores of Kohn) found between adjacent alveoli, permitting air to be distributed more evenly between them.

2. Diffusion

Diffusion is the process by which gases travel across the blood-gas interface in the alveolar-capillary network. A law of physiology states that the rate of gas transfer through a

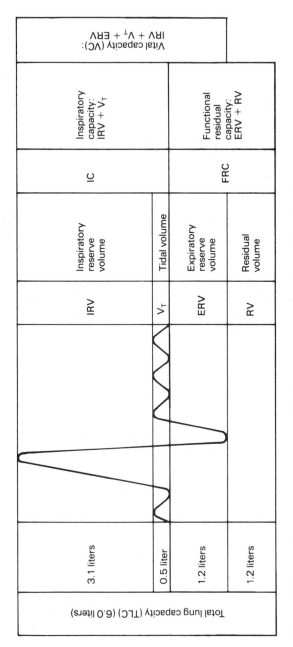

Figure 1-3 *Respiratory volumes and capacities. Inspiratory reserve volume (IRV) is the volume of air in a deep respiration. Expiratory reserve volume (ERV) is the volume of air in a full exhalation. Residual volume (RV) is the volume of air that remains in the lungs at all times.*

TABLE 1-1

SIGNIFICANCE OF PULMONARY FUNCTION VALUES

Pulmonary function test	Obstructive disease	Restrictive disease
Forced expiratory volume (1 sec.) (FEV_1)	↓	Normal
Vital capacity (VC)	Normal	↓
Functional residual capacity (FRC)	↑	↓ or normal
Total lung capacity (TLC)	↑ or normal	↓
Maximum midexpiratory flow rate (MMEFR)	↓	Normal
Maximum voluntary ventilation (MVV)	↓	Normal

sheet of tissue is proportional to the tissue area and the difference in gas concentration between the two sides, and inversely proportional to tissue thickness. Consequently, the alveolar-capillary membrane is ideal for diffusion because it has a large surface area (the size of a tennis court if the alveoli were spread out side by side) and the membrane is very thin. In healthy lungs, then, oxygen travels from alveolus to red blood cell without difficulty (see Figure 1-4).

The alveolar oxygen tension (PaO_2) approximately equals the arterial oxygen tension (PaO_2). However, this is not true in disease, and diffusion defects can cause hypoxemia. Carbon dioxide is also very diffusible; in fact, it is 20 times more diffusible than oxygen.

3. Perfusion

Perfusion is the actual blood flow through the pulmonary circulation. Since this is a low-pressure system, the pulmonary vasculature normally can vary its resistance to accommodate the blood flow it receives. The major factor affecting perfusion in the lung thus is cardiac output. This can be measured clinically with a pulmonary artery thermodilution catheter. As in the case of ventilation, blood flow is greater at the base of the lung than at the top (upright lung).

Figure 1-4 *The diffusion process. Reproduced, with permission, from Guyton AC: Textbook of Medical Physiology, 6th ed. Philadelphia: Saunders, 1981.*

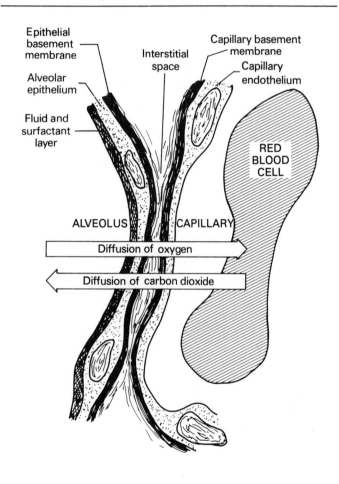

4. Ventilation/perfusion (V̇/Q̇) relationships

Gas exchange is most effective when there is a close match between lung ventilation and lung perfusion. In healthy lungs, the ventilation to perfusion ratio is 0.8. Any lung dysfunction will cause a significant mismatching of blood to gas, which leads to ineffective lung function. Mismatching may be due to either physiologic shunting, dead space, or both (see Figure 1-5).

a. Physiologic shunting. This occurs when perfusion exceeds ventilation in a given respiratory unit (alveolus and capillary). Such excess perfusion is called *venous admixture*, which means that some of the blood returns to the heart and to the rest of the body unoxygenated.

b. Physiologic dead space. This wasted ventilation occurs when there is ventilation but no perfusion to a respiratory unit (as when there is a pulmonary embolus). Anatomic dead space is the volume of air in conducting airways, and alveolar dead space is the volume of air in alveoli that are not perfused.

Figure 1-5 *Ventilation/perfusion relationships. Courtesy of the artist.*

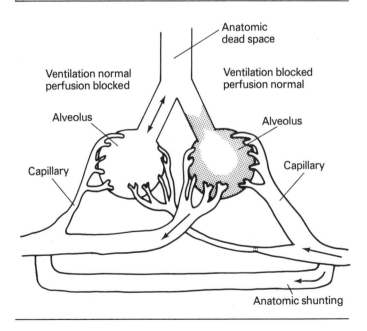

c. Ventilation-perfusion mismatching. This is the crux of lung pathophysiology and the reason for gas exchange problems in the lung. Such mismatching occurs slightly in healthy lungs because there is slightly more perfusion than ventilation. Mismatching, which increases in disease states, is due to one or more of the following relationships:

- Normal unit — ventilation and perfusion are relatively equal
- Dead space unit — alveoli are ventilated but not perfused
- Shunt unit — alveoli are perfused but not ventilated
- Silent unit — both alveolus and capillary are collapsed or blocked.

5. Oxygenation and oxygen transport

A major function of the lungs is to exchange carbon dioxide for oxygen and initiate oxygen transport via the circulation to the rest of the body. How well unoxygenated blood becomes oxygenated depends on P_aO_2, and how well oxygen is delivered to individual tissue cells depends on blood oxygen transport. Inability to oxygenate may lead to hypoxemia and/or hypoxia.

a. (P_aO_2). This is the major factor in oxygenating desaturated blood. It is determined by several factors:

- Fraction of inspired oxygen (F_iO_2) — the concentration of oxygen in the inhaled air; if the F_iO_2 increases, the P_aO_2 will also increase
- Alveolar gas exchange — the faster the rate of air exchange in and out of the alveoli, the more oxygen delivered to the alveoli per unit of time; to some extent, this is determined by respiratory rate
- Mixed venous oxygen content — the amount of oxygen in the pulmonary artery before it reaches the alveolar-capillary network; if the mixed venous oxygen content is low, there must be an increase in the respiratory rate, an increase in F_iO_2, or a decrease in blood flow in order to oxygenate the capillary bed adequately
- Distribution of ventilation — uneven distribution of ventilation with respect to perfusion is the most common clinical cause of hypoxemia responsive to oxygen therapy.

b. Blood oxygen transport. Once blood has been oxygenated in the pulmonary capillaries, its delivery to individual tissue cells throughout the body depends upon:

- Cardiac output – the amount of blood pumped by the heart in 1 minute
- Oxyhemoglobin dissociation curve – most oxygen in the blood is attached to the hemoglobin (Hb) molecule (a very small amount is dissolved in plasma); since Hb has a high affinity for O_2, Hb will tend to be saturated by O_2 – a relationship illustrated by the oxyhemoglobin dissociation curve, which determines the percentage of Hb saturation by O_2 for any given oxygen tension (P_aO_2) (see Figure 1-6); as long as the hemoglobin saturation is adequate, body tissues will receive an adequate supply of oxygen
- Relationship between oxygen saturation and oxygen tension – depends on normal cardiac output, hemoglo-

Figure 1-6 *Oxyhemoglobin dissociation curve. Reproduced, with permission, from Guyton AC: Textbook of Medical Physiology, 6th ed. Philadelphia: Saunders, 1981.*

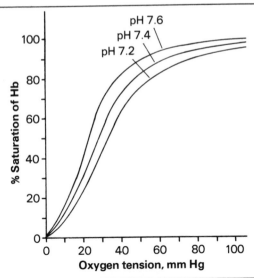

bin concentration, body temperature, and blood hydrogen ion concentration (pH)

- Hemoglobin-oxygen affinity—allows blood to oxygenate readily in the pulmonary capillary and determines relationship between O_2 saturation and O_2 tension in the oxyhemoglobin dissociation curve; a change in affinity can impair hemoglobin's ability to release O_2 to the tissues. Affinity itself is affected by carbon dioxide tension (P_aCO_2), temperature, pH, and 2,3-diphosphoglycerate (part of the enzyme system that regulates the affinity of hemoglobin for oxygen).

c. Hypoxemia (decreased P_aO_2). This is a decrease of oxygen tension in the arterial blood, and is not synonymous with hypoxia. Disorders leading to hypoxemia may be caused by low P_AO_2, primary alveolar hypoventilation (e.g., the impaired bellows mechanism in myasthenia gravis), $\dot{V}/\dot{Q}$ abnormalities (the most common cause—as in atelectasis, shock, pulmonary emboli), intrapulmonary shunting (as in adult respiratory distress syndrome [ARDS]), and diffusion defects (as in pulmonary fibrosis).

The lungs respond to hypoxemia by increasing the level of ventilation, via stimulation of the peripheral chemoreceptors. Increased ventilation (achieved by increasing the rate and/or depth of breathing) should then raise the P_aO_2, which would in turn elevate the blood oxygen tension. The most effective cardiovascular mechanism for correcting hypoxemia is to increase the cardiac output.

Only hypoxemia caused by a decrease in P_aO_2 will respond dramatically to oxygen therapy. Therefore, in venous admixture, where perfusion exceeds ventilation, oxygen therapy will be effective.

d. Hypoxia. This is a decrease of oxygen supplied to the tissues and occurs when critical cellular oxygen tensions are inadequate. With hypoxia, there is anaerobic metabolism which produces lactic acidemia. There are four types of hypoxia: hypoxic hypoxia—decreased P_aO_2; anemic hypoxia—decreased hemoglobin concentration; stagnant hypoxia—decreased cardiac output; and toxic hypoxia—

cyanide or carbon monoxide poisoning (prevents oxygen molecules from being delivered to cell).

6. Neurocontrol of ventilation

The rhythmicity of breathing is not inherent in the lung as it is in the heart. It is controlled by respiratory centers located in the brain.

a. Medulla. The inspiratory and expiratory centers located here control the rate and depth of ventilation to meet the body's metabolic demands.

b. Pons. The *apneustic center* (in the lower pons) stimulates the inspiratory medullary center and promotes deep, prolonged inspirations; and the *pneumotaxic center* (in the upper pons) stimulates the expiratory medullary center.

c. Receptor responses. Several groups of receptors assist the brain's control of respiratory function:

- *Central chemoreceptors* — located in the medulla, they respond to chemical changes in the cerebrospinal fluid, which are in turn due to chemical changes in the arterial blood; by responding to an increase in the pH, these receptors convey a message to the lungs to increase first the depth and then the rate of ventilation to correct the imbalance
- *Peripheral chemoreceptors* — located in the aortic arch and carotid arteries, these clusters of neurons respond first to P_aO_2, then to P_aCO_2 and pH
- *Hering-Breuer reflex* — these stretch receptors, located in the alveoli, become stimulated via the vagus nerve when the lungs are distended; therefore, inspiration is inhibited and there is no overdistention of the lungs
- *Proprioceptors in muscles and joints* — these receptors, which respond to body movements such as exercise, cause an increase in ventilation; thus, range of motion exercises for an immobile patient will stimulate breathing
- *Baroreceptors* — also located in the aortic and carotid bodies, these receptors respond to increased arterial blood pressure and cause reflex hypoventilation.

QUIZ

1. Identify whether the following lung structures are conducting or gas exchange airways:

Trachea _____

Alveolar sac _____

Bronchi _____

Respiratory bronchiole _____

Terminal bronchiole _____

Alveolar duct _____

2. On inspiration, the pressure within the lung becomes (positive/negative) relative to atmospheric pressure.

3. Surfactant is an important substance in the lung because it reduces _____, thereby preventing _____.

4. In each of the following conditions, identify whether there is predominantly inadequate perfusion (physiologic dead space) or inadequate ventilation (physiologic shunting):

Pulmonary embolus _____

Atelectasis _____

Pneumonia _____

Shock _____

5. True or false? Hypoxemia is caused by:

Low P_AO_2 _____

Alveolar hypoventilation _____

Low hemoglobin concentration _____

$\dot{V}/\dot{Q}$ abnormalities _____

6. The central chemoreceptors are located in the _____ and respond to changes in _____. The peripheral chemoreceptors are located in the _____ and respond to changes in _____.

ANSWERS

1. Trachea <u>conducting</u>.
Alveolar sac <u>gas exchange</u>.
Bronchi <u>conducting</u>.
Respiratory bronchiole <u>gas exchange</u>.
Terminal bronchiole <u>conducting</u>.
Alveolar duct <u>gas exchange</u>.

2. Negative.

3. Surface tension; atelectasis.

4. Pulmonary embolus <u>inadequate perfusion</u>.
Atelectasis <u>inadequate ventilation</u>.
Pneumonia <u>inadequate ventilation</u>.
Shock <u>inadequate perfusion</u>.

5. Low P_AO_2 <u>true</u>.
Alveolar hypoventilation <u>true</u>.
Low hemoglobin concentration <u>false</u>.
$\dot{V}/\dot{Q}$ abnormalities <u>true</u>.

6. Medulla, carbon dioxide tensions (P_aCO_2).
Carotid and aortic arches, oxygen tensions (P_aO_2).

Patient History

OBJECTIVES

After completing this chapter, you will be able to:

1. List the major elements of a respiratory history

2. Identify three major factors that contribute to lung disease.

A. Patient history in pulmonary disease

1. Why a history?

Rather quickly in a patient interview you can determine if the patient had, has, or is at high risk of developing a respiratory problem. The patient's history will relate to the physical findings and will often indicate why the patient has certain signs and symptoms. Although a complete medical history is important in caring for any patient, we'll focus here on those specific aspects of the history that relate to the respiratory system.

2. Acute versus chronic

First, it's important to differentiate (if possible) between an acute and a chronic condition. An acute problem will have recent physical findings that the patient will report. Usually an acute lung condition is related to a specific event (accident, exposure to an irritant, or recent cold) or else the signs and symptoms are fairly new. The patient with an acute problem typically has no underlying lung condition – just the findings associated with the acute episode.

Your questions should focus on the acute episode and on the complaints that led the patient to seek medical help. Be aware, though, that some patients have an acute problem on top of a chronic condition and that historical information must be obtained about each. If the patient has a chronic lung condition he can probably tell you his diagnosis, which may explain his particular findings. All histories you will obtain from patients with chronic pulmonary problems will be similar in cause, contributing factors, onset, signs, and symptoms.

B. Chief complaint

Whether the pulmonary problem is acute or chronic, the patient's complaint will probably relate to dyspnea, pain, shortness of breath, mucus, wheezing, swelling, cough, or general fatigue or weakness. Document what the patient (or accompanying friend or relative) sees as the major reason why he is seeking help.

C. Onset of illness

Find out when the chief complaint started, how long it lasted, and if it was relieved at any time and by what. Also, ask the patient when his general lung condition started, whether it has gotten progressively worse, and whether there is anything he does that makes him feel better. Make sure you obtain information on precipitating factors, duration, severity, and associated factors and/or symptoms (cough, mucus, fatigue, weight loss, diaphoresis, etc.).

D. Specific symptoms

The more specific information you can get about his problems, the more you will understand about his condition and the level of nursing care required.

1. Dyspnea

Remember that dyspnea is a symptom and therefore subjective. The patient will describe it the way he perceives it, which may or may not be consistent with the severity of his condition. Ask him about its onset, severity, and how much exercise he can perform easily. Ask about any difficulty getting air into or out of the lungs; if the patient purses his lips to breathe; and whether he sleeps better with several pillows under his head (orthopnea).

2. Chest pain

Determine the character of the pain. Since there are no nerve endings in the lung parenchyma, most chest pain will be cardiac in origin and its nature must be identified in detail. Pain due to a respiratory condition will arise from the pleura or respiratory muscles and ribs and is usually related to respirations. True chest pain needs to be distinguished from dyspnea, which the patient may describe as pain.

3. Cough

Ask the patient what causes him to cough, how long it lasts, and what relieves it. Find out if he coughs during a particular time of day and how many times a day he coughs. Ask him if the cough produces sputum, and (if so) whether it depends upon his body's position (upright or lying down) and if it is exhausting. Ask him if he has ever had a hernia or fractured a rib due to coughing.

4. Sputum

As in the case of coughing, the production of sputum always suggests an abnormality. Ask about the color, amount, consistency, and frequency of any sputum. Ask specifically if the patient coughs up either blood clots or blood-tinged sputum. Determine if there are any aggravating or alleviating factors.

E. Contributing factors

Several factors may contribute to lung conditions (especially chronic conditions).

1. Previous self or family history

Some conditions (asthma, emphysema) are due to previous lung problems (frequent infections, pneumonia, or kypho-scoliosis). Others arise because of a predisposing family history (asthma, alpha$_1$-antitrypsin deficiency).

2. Occupational history

In many industries people must work with substances that are now known to irritate the airways and can cause permanent lung damage or cancer. Any industry that emits smoke, dust, fumes, or chemical by-products should be suspect. Ask your patient about his past and present employment and how many years he has spent in what types of work. It's important to determine whether the patient's present condition can be traced back to a previous job.

3. Hobbies

Substances used in various hobbies can irritate the airways— for example, aerosol sprays, paints, or oils. Determine if any of these may be a contributing factor.

4. Allergens and environmental pollutants

Ask the patient if he has any known allergies (to dust, molds, pollens, foods, animals, drugs) and list them. If none is known, ask if he wheezes or experiences a shortness of breath at certain times of the year, at certain places, or during certain activities. There are many allergens that people may be exposed to at their places of work that cause lung diseases.

5. Smoking

The single most important factor that contributes to lung disease is cigarette smoking (but also cigar and pipe smoking). In taking a smoking history, find out how long the patient smoked, how many packs a day, and (if he has quit) how long since he stopped. If the patient is a child, find out if the parents smoke. If the patient does not smoke but works or lives in an environment where there is a lot of tobacco smoke, this may be a contributing factor.

F. Psychosocial and emotional factors

1. Stressors

Ask the patient about any stresses in his life such as anxiety, role change (job change), family relationships, financial problems, and employment/disability.

2. Coping mechanisms

Try to determine, either by observation or questioning the patient (or accompanying friend or relative), if he is reacting to problems in his life by means of anxiety, anger, hostility, dependency, withdrawal, isolation, avoidance, noncompliance, acceptance, or denial.

3. Support systems

Find out what support systems the patient could utilize to help him deal with his illness. Are there supportive family members, significant others, friends, community resources, or governmental resources available?

G. Sample history questionnaire

The sample questionnaire presented here (Figure 2-1) is particularly useful if the patient has a chronic illness. It can either be completed by the patient himself or be used as the basis for an interview.

Figure 2-1 *Patient history questionnaire*

Name _____

Date _____ Social Security number _____

Have you ever been told that you had:

	Yes	No	When	Nurse's comments
Tuberculosis				
Emphysema				
Bronchitis				
Asthma				
Pneumonia				
Flu				
High blood pressure				
Heart disease				

List any past hospitalizations. Be sure to include the date (year), the reason for hospitalization, and surgery if any was done.

_____

_____

_____

_____

List *all* the medications you are taking.

_____

_____

_____

Are you allergic to any medications? If so, list them.

_____

_____

Do you have any other allergies (food, pollens, molds, soaps)?

_____

_____

Do you use oxygen? _____

Do you use an IPPB machine? _____

Please check correct statement:

I usually cough:

_____ Only with colds or not at all

_____ Occasionally, but not on most days

_____ A little on most days

_____ A lot on most days

I raise chest mucus or sputum:

_____ Only with colds or not at all

_____ Occasionally, but not on most days

_____ In small amounts on most days

_____ In large amounts on most days

The raised sputum is:

_____ Usually white or clear

_____ Usually yellow or green or gray or brown

and

_____ Never colored with blood

_____ Only recently colored with blood

_____ For years colored with blood

My chest sounds wheezy or whistling:

_____ Only with colds or not at all

_____ Occasionally, but not on most days

_____ Only with physical exertion

_____ A lot on most days

My breathing is usually:

_____ Free and easy most of the time

_____ Slowing me down

_____ Keeping me close to home

_____ Keeping me mostly in one room

I wake during the night with trouble breathing:

_____ Never

_____ Occasionally

I sleep with:

_____ One or two pillows under my head

_____ Three or more pillows under my head

My feet, ankles, or legs:

_____ Never swell

_____ Swell some of the time

_____ Are usually swollen

Figure 2-1 (continued)

Have you ever smoked cigarettes?	____ Yes	____ No
If yes, at what age did you start smoking?		_____
Are you still smoking?	____ Yes	____ No
If yes, how many packs a day do you smoke?		_____
Have you ever wanted to stop smoking?		_____
If you have stopped, how old were you when you stopped?		_____
How many packs a day did you smoke?		_____
Are you on any special diet?	____ Yes	____ No

Have you ever been instructed in:

	No	Yes	When and where
Causes of lung diseases			
Breathing exercises			
Medications for lung disease			
Respiratory equipment			
Chest physical therapy			

Briefly describe what you do during a typical day. Begin with the time you usually wake up and end with your usual bedtime. For instance, include when and if you eat meals, get dressed, go outside of the house, watch TV, or do household chores.

What is the most difficult or discouraging thing that you must cope with as a person who has a lung condition?

QUIZ

1. In a respiratory history it is important to differentiate between _____ and _____ conditions.

2. List three specific symptoms often found in a patient with a respiratory condition:

3. List three factors that contribute to the development of lung disease:

4. What three psychosocial factors should be evaluated in a patient with lung disease?

ANSWERS

1. Acute; chronic.
2. Dyspnea, chest pain, cough.
3. Occupational history, smoking, allergies and environmental pollutants.
4. Stressors, coping mechanisms, support systems.

CHAPTER

3

Respiratory Assessment

OBJECTIVES

After completing this chapter, you will be able to:

1. List three physical findings you might observe in assessing the respiratory system by inspection

2. Evaluate lung expansion by palpation

3. Begin to differentiate between normal and adventitious breath sounds

4. Identify the voice sounds that may be heard in certain lung pathologies.

A. Introduction

A nursing assessment of all body systems is essential in order to establish a baseline of data about the patient and his condition. This information will facilitate detection of later changes and will serve as a reference point on the patient's status. But assessment is a dynamic process — it should be incorporated into all areas of nursing practice and patient care.

All patients entering the health care system ought to have a general nursing assessment. However, if the patient has a known or suspected pulmonary ailment, the respiratory system needs to be emphasized. Assessment should include inspection, palpation, percussion, and auscultation.

B. Inspection

Nurses probably perform this assessment better than anyone else in the health care system because of their ongoing contact with patients. Once a significant observation has been made, record it in writing and speak to the appropriate person about it. The following should be included in assessing the respiratory system:

1. General appearance

Several general observations can suggest that the patient either has a respiratory condition or is at high risk of developing one.

a. Body size. The obese patient is at risk because of the increased work load placed on his lungs to oxygenate a large amount of adipose tissue as well as the increased work of breathing required just to elevate the respiratory muscles in a fatty thorax. At the other extreme, the cachectic patient doesn't have much energy in reserve to meet the increased work of breathing that is required during any kind of illness.

b. Age. The very young and the very old are also at increased risk. The neonate (particularly the premature infant) may have problems due to incompletely developed lungs (respiratory distress syndrome), and the elderly may be at increased risk because, as part of the aging process, the lungs develop emphysematous changes with all of the typical signs and symptoms.

c. Skin quality. Notice the quality of the skin: What is its turgor (for evaluating hydration)? What is its temperature? Is the patient diaphoretic? If these findings are abnormal, there may be metabolic demands that will increase the body's need for oxygen and thus the work load of the lungs.

d. Posture. Now observe the patient's posture. How does he stand, sit, or lie down? A patient who has chronic difficulty in breathing will assume a posture that allows maximal elevation of the apex of the lungs and the intercostal muscles. If the patient leans against a wall while standing or rests his hands on a table or back of a chair in order to breathe, he is breathing inadequately. So, too, is the bedridden patient who leans forward with his hands on his knees or leans on a table placed in front of him. If the patient is extremely short of breath, he will not be able to lie horizontally and will keep the hospital bed in a semi-Fowler's or high-Fowler's position.

e. Chest configuration. Notice the external configuration of the chest — is the anterior-posterior diameter increased? That is, is the diameter from anterior to posterior as wide as (or wider than) the transverse diameter? If it is, then the patient probably has enlarged lung fields due to overinflated alveoli (as in emphysema). An extreme example of this would be the barrel chest. Look for other abnormalities of the chest, which could suggest underlying lung impairment (see Table 3-1).

f. Mentation. If a patient is anxious, apprehensive, restless, confused, drowsy, lethargic, or comatose, or demonstrates a dramatic personality change, hypoxia or hypercapnia must be considered. Headaches, especially at night or early morning, in someone with a chronic respiratory condition suggest hypercapnia.

TABLE 3-1

ABNORMAL CHEST CONFIGURATIONS

Finding	*Reason*
Increased A-P diameter	Overinflated alveoli
Pectus excavatum (funnel chest)	Congenital (may compromise CP status)
Pectus carinatum (pigeon breast)	Congenital
Scars	Lobectomy, pneumonectomy, heart surgery
Kyphosis	Chronically compresses chest expansion
Scoliosis	Chronically compresses chest expansion

2. Skin color

The sign usually associated with breathing problems is cyanosis; it is a very late indication of hypoxia. In order for cyanosis to appear, there must be a drop of 5 gm/100 ml of oxygenated hemoglobin (Hb). A patient whose Hb is 15 gm/100 ml will not demonstrate cyanosis until 5 gm/100 ml of that Hb becomes unoxygenated, resulting in an effective circulating Hb of two-thirds the normal level. This is true even if the patient's usual level of Hb is 5 gm or 25 gm/100 ml, and so the presence of cyanosis is not a reliable sign (the anemic patient will die before cyanosis appears, and the polycythemic patient will always look cyanotic but will be adequately oxygenated).

In trying to observe cyanosis, take into consideration the room lighting, skin color, and depth of the vessels from the surface of the skin, for these factors will affect skin color. In the presence of a pulmonary condition, look for central cyanosis by observing the color of the tongue and lips (this indicates a decrease in oxygen tension in the blood). Peripheral cyanosis — decreased blood flow to a certain area of the body (as in vasoconstriction of the nailbeds and ear lobes due to cold weather) — does not necessarily indicate a central systemic problem.

3. Characteristics of respirations

It is not sufficient to look at a patient's chest and simply count respirations. You can learn a great deal about the patient's respiratory status by observing the way he breathes. First, identify which muscles are being used for ventilation; the most effective ones are the diaphragm, the intercostals, and the abdominal muscles. If the patient is using his accessory (e.g., sternocleidomastoid) muscles, is demonstrating substernal or excessive intercostal retractions or paradoxical abdominal muscle movements (the abdomen sucks in on inspiration and pushes out on expiration), he will have labored respirations because of the increased work of breathing.

Ask the patient if he has air hunger or is short of breath; if so, you will know he is dyspneic (since dyspnea is subjective, only the patient can identify this symptom). Pursed lip breathing (exhaling through pursed lips) may also be seen in some patients who are extremely short of breath. Try to determine the severity of the dyspnea by asking the patient what activity causes him to be short of breath, how long it lasts, and what he does to get his breath back.

While examining the chest, check to see if there is equal expansion of both sides and if there is movement of all lungs fields. If there is chest trauma, look carefully for a flail chest (paradoxical chest movement in a specific area due to a fracture of several ribs on one side, a fracture of the sternum, or a rib that is fractured in at least two places, producing an unstable chest wall).

As you are counting respirations (in someone with altered respiratory status, respirations should be counted for a full minute, rather than the conventional 15 seconds), try to determine if the patient has a specific pattern of breathing (see Table 3-2).

4. Cough and secretions

Being able to observe the patient's cough and secretions is helpful in determining the presence of infection or in evaluating the patient's ability to handle his own secretions. However, if you cannot observe him coughing, you may have

TABLE 3-2

PATTERNS OF BREATHING

Apnea	Absent breath sounds
Eupnea	Normal breathing: 12-18 breaths per minute
Tachypnea	Rapid breathing: more than 22 breaths per minute
Bradypnea	Slow breathing: fewer than 10 breaths per minute
Hyperventilation	Increased rate and/or depth of breathing, causing P_aCO_2 to fall below normal
Hypoventilation	Underventilation, causing P_aCO_2 to rise above normal
Orthopnea	Patient must sit up to breathe
Dyspnea on exertion (DOE)	Shortness of breath during activity
Paroxysmal nocturnal dyspnea (PND)	Shortness of breath while sleeping or resting
Cheyne-Stokes respiration	Progressive increase in volume followed by progressive decrease in volume of each breath until a period of apnea occurs
Stertorous breathing	Snoring caused by relaxation of the soft palate or secretions in the upper respiratory tract
Stridor	Inspiratory shrill caused by constriction or spasm of upper airway
Dyspnea	Shortness of breath

to rely on the patient's history. (The patient may not be able to give an accurate report of his coughing, however, because coughing has become an accepted social phenomenon nowadays with the prevalence of smoking.)

Coughing is a reflex mechanism that helps keep the lungs free of foreign matter (smoke, physical agents, irritants, microorganisms, etc.) (see Figure 3-1). The presence of a cough, then, indicates that something is abnormal and that the body is trying to correct the problem. Although it is an essential defense mechanism, coughing may be so weak that it is ineffective (as in the debilitated or postoperative patient) or it may be so violent that it is exhausting (and can even cause a fractured rib). Therefore, it is important to

Figure 3-1 *Cough reflex. Reproduced, with permission, from Cherniack RM: Respiration in Health and Disease, ed 2. Philadelphia, WB Saunders, 1972, p 169.*

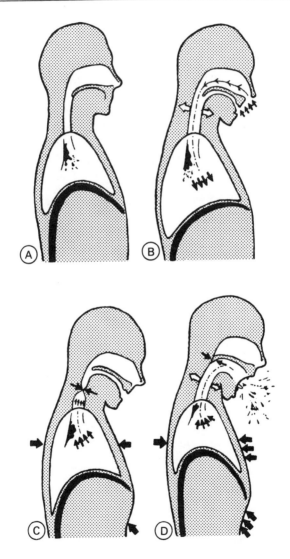

A. Irritation. B. Inspiration. C. Compression. D. Expulsion.

evaluate the presence or absence of coughing, its effectiveness, and its frequency.

Coughing is usually associated with accumulated secretions. Adults normally produce about 100 ml of mucus a day, but this is not seen because it is absorbed by the lymphatics, swallowed, or ingested by macrophages in the alveoli. Therefore, the expectoration of mucus is always abnormal; if mucus cannot be handled in the usual way, either it is coughed up or it accumulates in the lung. Damaged cilia also make it more difficult for the lung to handle mucus. If mucus is present, observe and document the amount, consistency, and color (all may be signs of infection).

5. Clubbing

Clubbing exists when the base angle between the nail and the nailbed is either flat (180 degrees) or greater than 180 degrees. The mechanism of clubbing is unclear, but it occurs in advanced COPD. Although it develops slowly and is not treated, it suggests pathology. Be aware, though, that clubbing is also found in congenital heart disease and liver disease.

6. Vital signs

Although vital signs are not an observation skill, they are an integral part of a respiratory assessment, for they can indicate respiratory problems.

C. Palpation

This is the act of feeling the chest to delineate areas of pain, masses, and consolidation, and to evaluate the degree of expansion. Palpating chest expansion is a more sensitive indicator than just inspecting expansion. The technique calls for placing your hands flat on the chest wall (palms down) with your thumbs meeting in the middle (sternum anteriorly and the spine posteriorly) during end-expiration. Ask the patient to take a deep breath; your thumbs will swing out with the chest freely while your other fingers remain on the chest wall as it expands (see Figure 3-2). Then ask the patient to exhale, allowing your thumbs to come together again.

If your thumbs move equally in all lung areas, this is called bilateral chest expansion. But if one thumb does not move as much as the other (unilateral expansion), this may indicate lung mass, lung abscess, atelectasis, pneumothorax, or emphysematous blebs on the affected side.

Vocal and tactile fremitus should also be assessed by palpation. To elicit vocal fremitus, place your hand (palm down) flat on the patient's chest. Then ask the patient to say "99." In the normal, healthy chest, this is readily felt as vibrations on the fingertips. If the vibrations are diminished or absent, this may indicate pleural effusion, thickened pleura, pneumonia, or atelectasis.

Tactile fremitus is achieved simply by placing your hand flat on the patient's chest wall as he breathes (without vocalizing). If you feel vibrations during inspiration or expiration, this indicates the movement of liquid with air flow (which occurs in consolidation or other conditions where rhonchi can be heard on auscultation).

Figure 3-2 *Palpation for chest expansion*

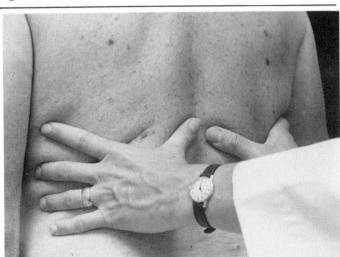

D. Percussion

This is the act of striking the surface of the body to elicit a sound so that the underlying tissue can be evaluated. As an assessment skill, percussion of the chest requires more practice to develop than does inspection or palpation. The most popular way to do it is to place the middle finger of your left hand (if you are right-handed) on the patient's chest and strike the distal phalanx of this finger with the tip of the middle finger of your right hand (Figure 3-3). The blow should be short, sharp, staccato, and rhythmic, struck as quickly and as hard as possible.

The sound produced is determined by the density of the underlying tissue. However, it is a subtle sound and cannot easily be evaluated in a noisy environment. Generally

Figure 3-3 *Percussion technique*

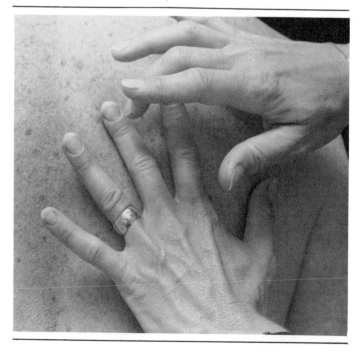

speaking, a hollow percussion sound means that the underlying tissue contains air (as in the normal lung), while a dull to flat sound suggests a solid piece of tissue (as in the thigh or kidney). Practice percussion by listening for the following sounds in the corresponding body parts: tympanic (cheek filled with air), hyperresonance (air in empty stomach), resonance (lung), dull (kidney), and flat (thigh).

The posterior lung should be percussed first, starting at the apices and alternating between the right and left lungs. If there is a specific area of density (as in the heart anteriorly), this should also be outlined via percussion. After you have percussed down to the bases of the posterior chest, percuss the anterior chest in the same way. Make sure that the finger is struck in the intercostal space with each hand placement. This will ensure a better evaluation of the sound since the percussion then will not have to go through bone.

On percussion, the normal chest produces a hollow or resonant sound in all lung fields. A hyperresonant or tympanic sound suggests a pneumothorax or emphysematous blebs. A dull or flat sound suggests an area of consolidation with exudate, atelectasis, neoplasm, or pleural effusion. Of course, percussion alone cannot identify a specific problem; it must be combined with other assessment techniques as well as laboratory data and chest X-ray.

E. Auscultation

Here, the stethoscope is used to listen to the sound produced in the lung as air passes in and out of the airways. The binaural stethoscope has two chestpieces. The diaphragm chestpiece is the larger, flat piece covered with a Bakelite filter, which filters out low-pitched sounds so that high-pitched sounds can be heard well. Since the diaphragm chestpiece is intended for general screening, it is used to listen to blood pressure, bowel sounds, bruits, normal heart sounds, and breath sounds. The bell chestpiece is a smaller, concave piece used mainly to detect abnormal heart sounds such as clicks and murmurs. Remember that the stethoscope only transmits sound; it does not amplify or augment the sound in any way.

The preferred technique for auscultating the chest is to begin with the patient sitting upright and breathing deeply in and out through the mouth. Using the diaphragm chestpiece, listen to the apices of the anterior chest, alternating from one lung to the other. The best way to detect abnormalities is to compare an affected area with the same spot in the contralateral lung. Traverse the anterior chest down to the anterior bases of the lung. Then listen posteriorly, starting at the apices and zigzagging across the chest, working down to the bases.

This method can be time-consuming and may not be realistic for busy, practicing nurses. If so, in the initial assessment, auscultate the patient's anterior chest, listening to one area in each lobe (unless an abnormal finding necessitates further exploration) for a total of six positions anteriorly. Then, when the patient is turned for the first time, use this opportunity to listen to the posterior chest in a sampling of six spots (see Figure 3-4). Pay special attention to the posterior bases, for that is where fluid and secretions tend to accumulate by gravity in a semirecumbent patient. A word of caution: If the patient's condition suggests that there may be abnormal findings in the initial assessment (e.g., the patient with repeated episodes of congestive heart failure [CHF]), auscultate the posterior lung right away.

In order to evaluate breath sounds effectively, you must listen to the bare chest, as clothing of any kind may produce a rubbing sound that falsely mimics rales. If possible, the patient should sit upright and should breathe slowly and deeply through the mouth (normal breaths through the nose do not usually generate enough air flow to produce sound). Take care that the patient does not become light-headed from hyperventilation. If a rales-like sound is heard in a very hairy-chested patient, you may need to wet the hairs to reduce the friction between them and the stethoscope.

Sound is produced when air is made to vibrate as it passes through the airways in the lung. The sounds heard are characterized by their duration, pitch, intensity (or amplitude), and timbre (or quality). Figure 3-5 shows a method of diagramming breath sounds.

Figure 3-4 *Auscultation sequence*

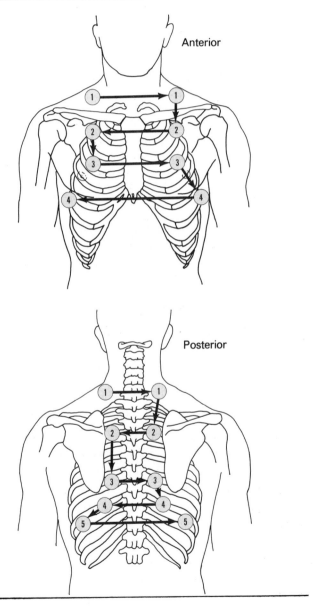

Figure 3-5 *Depiction of breath sounds*

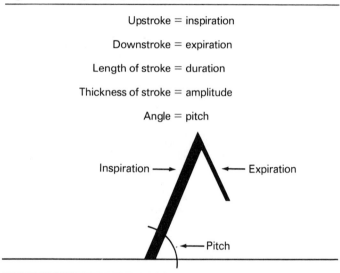

Upstroke = inspiration

Downstroke = expiration

Length of stroke = duration

Thickness of stroke = amplitude

Angle = pitch

Inspiration → ← Expiration

← Pitch

1. Normal breath sounds

a. Vesicular. Produced by air moving through alveoli in all peripheral lung fields (Figure 3-6), the smooth "swishing" sound resembles that of air whistling through the trees. The sound is heard mainly on inspiration, because air flow is more forceful at that time than on expiration. This sound is usually documented as "lungs clear."

b. Harsh vesicular. A sound of increased intensity and duration, this occurs in children because of their thin, elastic chest wall, and also following vigorous exercise.

c. Diminished vesicular. A sound of decreased intensity and duration, this occurs in the elderly with rigid, inelastic chest walls; in the obese and muscular; and in certain pathologic states, such as emphysema.

d. Bronchial (tubular). Produced as air moves through large airways (the trachea and bronchi), bronchial sounds are heard over the manubrium sterni and the lower part of the trachea (Figure 3-6). The expiration sound is louder and longer than that of inspiration, and there is a "silent gap" between the two phases. The bronchial breath sound is coarser and harsher than the vesicular because it comes from the largest airways. When heard in the lung parenchyma, it becomes an abnormal breath sound and denotes disease.

Figure 3-6 *Normal breath sounds and their locations*

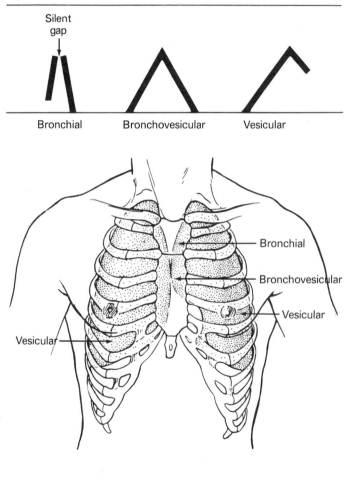

e. Bronchovesicular. This combination of bronchial and vesicular sounds is produced as air moves through large airways and alveolar tissue. It is heard over the sternum anteriorly and between the scapulae posteriorly (Figure 3-6). The sound is louder and harsher than vesicular breath sounds, but not as loud or as coarse as bronchial. Inspiration and expiration have equal weight, and there is no pause between the phases.

2. Abnormal breath sounds

a. Diminished or absent. If this is what you detect in any lung field, first make sure that the stethoscope is working and that the patient took a deep breath. No sound is heard when there is decreased or absent air flow to an area of the lung, as in the case of tumors, atelectasis, pneumothorax, paralyzed diaphragm, emphysematous blebs, adipose tissue, or malpositioned endotracheal tube.

b. Bronchial. When heard in the lung parenchyma, these sounds mean that the alveoli in the area are filled with fluid or exudate, and so air does not flow through them. These sounds resemble normal bronchial sounds heard in the lower trachea. However, when abnormal, these sounds can be caused by pneumonia, atelectasis, secretions, tumors not obstructing a bronchus, shock lung, or pleural effusion.

3. Adventitious breath sounds

a. Rales. These are popping, crackling, discontinuous, non-musical noises heard mainly on inspiration (Figure 3-7). They are believed to be caused by (1) alveoli that are closed at end-expiration and then pop open again with the next inspiration, or (2) air popping through fluid in the alveoli. Rales indicate small airways or alveolar disease and can be heard in pulmonary edema, pneumonia, TB, interstitial fibrosis, and COPD.

b. Rhonchi. There are two types of rhonchi, but both indicate disease in the large airways and are typically heard on expiration. One type is coarse rales that sound liquid and bubbly (Figure 3-7). The other consists of low-pitched wheezes and sounds like snoring, groaning, or moaning. Both types are

Figure 3-7 *Adventitious breath sounds*

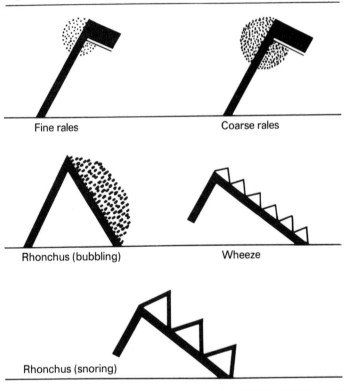

Fine rales

Coarse rales

Rhonchus (bubbling)

Wheeze

Rhonchus (snoring)

due to secretions or fluid as well as narrowing of the large airways; they may be heard in bronchitis, bronchiectasis, poor secretion removal (as in a postoperative or comatose patient), resolving pneumonia, or COPD.

c. Wheezes. These are high-pitched, squeaky, continuous, musical noises that sound like whistling or violins tuning up (Figure 3-7). Caused by a narrowing, constriction, or spasm of the small airways, they are most often heard on expiration (but can be heard anywhere in the breathing cycle). Wheezes occur in such conditions as asthma, COPD, pulmonary edema, pulmonary embolus, and pneumonia.

4. Voice sounds

These are not sounds produced by air moving through the airways, but a means of listening to the voice as it travels through the chest, thereby permitting evaluation of the underlying tissue.

a. Normal. The *normal* voice sound is produced in the larynx and then travels through the tracheobronchial tree to the alveoli and chest wall. When the patient says the test word "99," the sound heard through the chest wall is normally softer and less distinct (or more muffled) than when heard externally through the air.

b. Bronchophony. This occurs when the patient says "99" and the sound comes through the chest wall distinctly, clearly, and loudly. Bronchophony can be heard over areas of the lung where the alveoli are either filled with fluid or

TABLE 3-3

CLINICAL APPLICATION OF PULMONARY ASSESSMENT

Condition	Pathophysiologic description	Palpation (including fremitus)
Normal	Tracheobronchial tree and alveoli are open and clear; lung bellows mechanism intact; no respiratory effort or awareness	Bilateral expansion Normal fremitus
Atelectasis	A collapsed or atelectatic lung due to insufficient volume to keep alveoli open and bronchial obstruction	Poor expansion in affected area if severe; decreased or absent tactile and vocal fremitus
Pneumonia (pulmonary consolidation)	Bronchi open but contain secretions; alveoli are filled with fluid, red and white cells	Normal expansion, increased vocal and tactile fremitus
COPD Bronchitis	Bronchial irritation, inflammation; increased secretions	Normal expansion; tactile and vocal fremitus increased

replaced by solid tissue. It is heard in the same conditions that produce bronchial breath sounds (i.e., pneumonia, atelectasis, tumors).

c. Whispered pectoriloquy. This occurs when the patient *whispers* "99" and the sound comes through loudly, clearly, distinctly, and intelligibly. It has the same significance and occurs in the same conditions as bronchophony, but it is more sensitive.

d. Egophony. When the patient says "e," egophony is present the sound heard through the chest wall changes to "a." It is a loud, nasal sound that can be heard above a pleural effusion or abscess and sometimes over a consolidated lung.

A summary of the assessment findings in various conditions is presented in Table 3-3.

Percussion note	Voice sounds	Breath sounds	Adventitious breath sounds
Resonant	Normal	Vesicular with bronchovesicular near large bronchi	None
Dull	Decreased to absent	Decreased vesicular or absent	None (rales if secretion-related)
Dull	Increased bronchophony, whispered pectoriloquy, possibly egophony	Bronchial (tubular)	Rales and rhonchi
Resonant	None	Normal to bronchial	Wheezes, rhonchi, or rales

TABLE 3-3 (continued)

Condition	Pathophysiologic description	Palpation (including fremitus)
Asthma	Increased mucosal edema, bronchospasm and mucus production	Increased tactile and vocal fremitus
Emphysema	Overinflated alveoli; destruction of alveolar septa; bronchioles close too soon from loss of elastic recoil; results in increased mucus, decreased cilia function, trapping of air, poor gas exchange	Flattened diaphragm; ↑ AP diameter; minimal expansion bilaterally; tactile and vocal fremitus decreased
Pneumothorax	Interruption of negative pleural pressure results in collapsed lung and loss of integrity of bellows mechanism	Pain, little or no expansion on affected side. Trachea shifted to opposite side in tension pneumothorax; decreased tactile and vocal fremitus
Misplaced endotracheal tube	Tube in right mainstem bronchus results in no expansion, ventilation and exchange of left lung, and eventual collapse	No expansion on affected side; may have deviated trachea
Pulmonary edema	Interstitial fluid in small airways (alveoli and small bronchioles)	Normal; tactile or vocal fremitus may be slightly increased
ARDS	Leaky capillaries; destruction of alveolar membrane; loss of surfactant; congestive atelectasis; widened alveolar-capillary membrane; results in noncardiogenic pulmonary edema	Normal or poor bilateral expansion

Percussion note	Voice sounds	Breath sounds	Adventitious breath sounds
Resonant	None	Normal to bronchial. Short inspiration	Wheezes, rhonchi, or rales
Hyper-resonant	None	Prolonged expiration. Decreased vesicular	None to rales, rhonchi, or wheezes
Hyper-resonant	Decreased or absent	Decreased or absent	None
Hyper-resonant on affected side	Decreased or absent	Absent on affected side	None
Normal	Normal	Normal	Rales over both lung bases, sometimes wheezes
Normal	Normal	Bronchial	Rales, rhonchi, wheezes

QUIZ

1. Match the definition with the appropriate pattern of breathing:

Absence of
breathing _____

a. Eupnea

Rapid respirations _____

b. Apnea

Slow respirations _____

c. Tachypnea

Difficult breathing during
activity _____

d. Bradypnea

e. Orthopnea

Normal breathing _____

f. Dyspnea on exertion

Must sit up to
breathe _____

2. In a pleural effusion, pneumonia, or atelectasis, the vibrations produced during vocal fremitus are generally _____ .

3. Match the percussion sound heard with the lung condition that might produce it:

Emphysematous
blebs _____

a. Resonance

b. Hyperresonance

Normal chest _____

c. Dull

Pneumonia _____

4. Breath sounds are created as air is made to _____ in the air passages.

5. The normal breath sound heard in the peripheral lung fields is called _____ .

6. A harsher sound heard over the sternum and lower trachea is called _____ .

7. Match the breath sound most likely to be heard in the following conditions:

Congestive heart failure _____   **a.** Diminished sound

Bronchopneumonia _____   **b.** Wheezes

Asthma _____   **c.** Rales

Atelectasis _____   **d.** Rhonchi

8. Match the following conditions with the voice sounds that may be heard:

Bronchophony _____   **a.** Pneumonia

Whispered pectoriloquy _____   **b.** Pleural effusion

Egophony _____

ANSWERS

1. Absence of breathing **b**.
   Rapid respirations **c**.
   Slow respirations **d**.
   Difficult breathing during activity **f**.
   Normal breathing **a**.
   Must sit up to breathe **e**.

2. Diminished.

3. Emphysematous blebs **b**.
   Normal chest **a**.
   Pneumonia **c**.

4. Vibrate.

5. Vesicular.

6. Bronchial.

7. Congestive heart failure **c**.
   Bronchopneumonia **d**.
   Asthma **b**.
   Atelectasis **a**.

8. Bronchophony **a**.
   Whispered pectoriloquy **a**.
   Egophony **b**.

4

Arterial Blood Gas Interpretation

OBJECTIVES

After completing this chapter, you will be able to:

1. *Identify the acid-base disorder when you receive arterial blood gas (ABG) results*

2. *List two causes for respiratory acidosis, respiratory alkalosis, metabolic acidosis, and metabolic alkalosis*

3. *Determine if compensation is present when you are given an acid-base problem*

4. *List the three parameters measured by ABGs.*

A. Why arterial blood gases?

The major functions of the lung are oxygenation and ventilation, both of which play a role in maintaining the body's acid-base balance. In order to evaluate the oxygenation, ventilation, or acid-base balance status of your patient, you need to obtain ABG measurements. ABGs are drawn from an artery (usually radial, brachial, or femoral) into a special heparinized syringe, which is then analyzed. Once you have performed an arterial puncture, you must apply pressure to the site for approximately 5 minutes to make sure the artery stops bleeding completely.

B. Normal values

Table 4-1 gives the symbols, definitions, and normal ranges for arterial blood gases.

C. Acid-base balance

1. pH

The body is always striving to maintain a balance between acids and bases. Whether or not this is accomplished is indicated by the pH of the blood, representing the negative logarithm of the hydrogen ion concentration. The higher the hydrogen ion concentration, the more acid there is, and thus the lower the pH value. The lower the hydrogen ion concentration, the greater the amount of base (or alkali), and thus the higher the pH value. Consequently, pH < 7.35 indicates acidosis, and pH > 7.45 indicates alkalosis.

A normal pH must be maintained in order for each cell to function properly. Severe acidosis or alkalosis results in death if not treated (quiz question 5).

2. Three main body defenses

a. Buffers. These body substances are constantly trying to maintain acid-base balance by acting on acids and bases. The major buffer system is the relationship between bicarbonate ion (HCO_3^-) and carbonic acid (H_2CO_3). This relation-

RESPIRATORY PROBLEMS

ship is depicted in the Henderson-Hasselbalch equation, which is simplified as follows:

$$pH = \underset{\text{(constant)}}{pk} + \frac{HCO_3^- \text{ (base)}}{H_2CO_3 \text{ (acid)}}$$

Their relationship works as follows:

$$\text{Lung} \qquad\qquad \text{Kidney}$$
$$CO_2 \leftarrow CO_2 + H_2O \Leftrightarrow H_2CO_3 \Leftrightarrow H^+ + HCO_3^- \rightarrow \begin{array}{c} HCO_3^- \\ \text{or} \\ H^+ \end{array}$$

The body is constantly moving its buffers from one side of the equation to the other, depending on the need at any moment, in order to maintain a proper relationship between carbonic acid and bicarbonate ion. Three other buffers — phosphates, hemoglobin, and protein — help to maintain acid-base balance in the body, but to a lesser extent than bicarbonate and carbonic acid.

b. Lungs. The lungs control the hydrogen ion concentration, and therefore, the acid-base balance in the body, by varying
Continued on page 62

TABLE 4-1

NORMAL ARTERIAL BLOOD GAS VALUES

Symbol	Definition	Normal range
pH	Negative logarithm of hydrogen ion concentration in arterial blood	7.35-7.45
P_aO_2	Partial pressure of oxygen in arterial blood	80-100 mm Hg
P_aCO_2	Partial pressure of carbon dioxide in arterial blood	35-45 mm Hg
HCO_3^-	Bicarbonate ion (level of base in arterial blood)	22-28 mEq/liter
BE	Base excess (difference between acid and base levels in arterial blood)	−2 to +2 mEq/liter
S_aO_2	Saturation of hemoglobin by oxygen	>95%

TABLE 4-2

ACID-BASE DISORDERS

Disorder	Definition	Lab values	Causes

Respiratory acidosis	$\downarrow$ pH
	$\uparrow P_aCO_2$
		pH < 7.35
		$P_aCO_2 > 45$
		HCO_3^- or
		BE—normal
			Hypoventilation:
			  COPD
			  Neuromuscular
			    disease
			  Pneumonia with
			    secretions
			  Trauma
			  Oversedation
			  Anesthesia
			  Drug overdose

Respiratory alkalosis	$\uparrow$ pH
	$\downarrow P_aCO_2$
		pH > 7.45
		$P_aCO_2 < 35$
		HCO_3^- or
		BE—normal
			Emotions:
			  Anxiety
			  Anger
			  Hysteria
			Pain
			Hypoxia:
			  CHF
			  Pulmonary
			    embolus
			  Pulmonary
			    fibrosis
			  Brain trauma
			  Fever
			  Mechanical
			    ventilation

Metabolic acidosis	$\downarrow$ pH
	$\downarrow HCO_3^-$
	  or BE
		pH < 7.35
		P_aCO_2—
		  normal
		$HCO_3^- < 22$
		  or
		  BE < −2
			Diabetes
			Renal failure
			Lactic acidosis
			Diarrhea
			Hyperkalemia

Metabolic alkalosis	$\uparrow$ pH
	$\uparrow HCO_3^-$
	  or BE
		pH > 7.45
		P_aCO_2—
		  normal
		$HCO_3^- > 28$
		  or
		  BE > +2
			Vomiting, NG
			  suctioning
			Diuretics
			Antacids
			Some diarrhea
			Hypokalemia
			Hyperaldosteronism
			Hypochloremia

Clinical signs	Compensation	Medical treatment
↓ Ventilation Headache Sensorium changes: 　Irritability 　Impaired 　　judgment 　Semicomatose- 　　comatose Tachycardia Arrhythmias	pH — normal $P_aCO_2 > 45$ $HCO_3^- > 28$ or BE > +2	Treat cause Improve ventilation: 　IPPB, antibiotics 　Postural drainage 　Suctioning 　Incentive spirometry 　Ventilator HCO_3- in emergency
Tachypnea Numbness Tingling of hands 　and face Sensorium changes	pH—normal $P_aCO_2 < 35$ $HCO_3^- < 22$ or BE < —2	Treat cause Sedation Voluntary breath holding Oxygen 　↓ Ventilator setting
Headache Nausea, vomiting Diarrhea Sensorium changes Tremors Convulsions	pH—normal $P_aCO_2 < 35$ $HCO_3^- < 22$ or BE < —2	Treat underlying cause Give insulin in diabetes Dialyze if renal failure Give HCO_3- if necessary
Nausea, vomiting NG drainage Diarrhea Tremors Convulsions	pH—normal $P_aCO_2 > 45$ $HCO_3^- > 28$ or BE > +2	Replace loss of fluids Give K^+, Cl^- as needed Stop NG suctioning Give acidifying substances 　Arginine HCl 　HCl 　Ammonium Cl^-

the amount of CO_2 exhaled (see Equation 2). This response occurs within minutes of the body's need.

c. Kidneys. The kidneys regulate the acid-base balance by varying the excretion or reabsorption of hydrogen and bicarbonate ions (see Equation 2). This mechanism takes hours to adjust to the body's need.

3. Acid-base disorders

a. Respiratory acidosis ($\downarrow$pH, $\uparrow$$P_aCO_2$). If there is a condition that causes the lungs to retain CO_2, more acid will be formed in the body and the result will be respiratory acidosis. P_aCO_2 represents the level of ventilation; when it is increased in disease, the patient is hypoventilating. Conditions that cause hypoventilation can result in respiratory acidosis (see Table 4-2).

b. Respiratory alkalosis ($\uparrow$pH, $\downarrow$$P_aCO_2$). This is the opposite of respiratory acidosis. Now the patient is hyperventilating and blowing off excess CO_2. Since this results in less CO_2 available to combine with water, less acid is produced. Conditions that precipitate hyperventilation cause respiratory alkalosis (see Table 4-2; quiz questions 6 and 7).

c. Metabolic acidosis ($\downarrow$pH, $\downarrow$$HCO_3^-$ or $\downarrow$BE). To determine if the acidosis is caused by a metabolic problem, we evaluate the HCO_3^- or BE. This will indicate the amount of bicarbonate (or base) present in relation to the amount of acid. If the HCO_3^- or BE is decreased, there is excessive acid in relation to base, which the kidneys can't handle. Conditions that prevent the kidneys from getting rid of H+ or reabsorbing HCO_3^- or that produce more acid than the kidneys can handle lead to metabolic acidosis (see Table 4-2).

d. Metabolic alkalosis ($\uparrow$pH, $\uparrow$$HCO_3^-$ or $\uparrow$BE). In metabolic alkalosis, the HCO_3^- or BE is increased in relation to the amount of acid in the body. Either too much base is being produced in the body or too much acid is being removed. Conditions that cause either of these lead to metabolic alkalosis (see Table 4-2; quiz question 8).

4. Compensation for acid-base disorders

The body tries to re-establish normal pH by changing the system not primarily affected (see Table 4-3).

a. Respiratory acidosis. The kidneys reabsorb more bicarbonate or excrete more H^+, thereby raising the bicarbonate or BE level.

b. Respiratory alkalosis. The kidneys excrete more bicarbonate, thereby lowering the pH toward normal and decreasing the bicarbonate level.

c. Metabolic acidosis. The lungs hyperventilate to lower the CO_2 level; this raises the pH toward normal and decreases the P_aCO_2.

d. Metabolic alkalosis. The lungs retain CO_2 by lowering the rate of ventilation; this decreases the pH and increases the P_aCO_2 (see quiz question 9).

5. Medical correction

If the body's own compensatory mechanisms cannot function effectively, we can correct the situation medically by treating the system that is primarily affected (see Table 4-2).

a. Respiratory acidosis. Increase and assist ventilation.

TABLE 4-3

HOW THE BODY COMPENSATES FOR ACID-BASE DISTURBANCES

Disturbance	Abnormality			Compensation		
	pH	P_aCO_2	HCO_3^-	pH	P_aCO_2	HCO_3^-
Metabolic acidosis	↓	N	↓	Near N	↓	↓
Metabolic alkalosis	↑	N	↑	Near N	↑	↑
Respiratory acidosis	↓	↑	N	Near N	↑	↑
Respiratory alkalosis	↑	↓	N	Near N	↓	↓
Mixed acidosis	↓	↑	↓	Not possible		
Mixed alkalosis	↑	↓	↑	Not possible		

N = normal.

b. Respiratory alkalosis. Decrease or stop hyperventilation.

c. Metabolic acidosis. Give bicarbonate or treat the cause of acid accumulation or bicarbonate loss.

d. Metabolic alkalosis. Give arginine HCl, HCl, KCl, NH₄Cl, or fluids.

QUIZ

1. The status of what three parameters can be evaluated with an ABG?

2. What acid-base disturbance do the following ABG values indicate? pH—7.29, P_aO_2—80, P_aCO_2—55, HCO_3^-—24?

3. For each of the following conditions, what is the acid-base disturbance?

Diabetes _____	**a.** Respiratory acidosis
Vomiting _____	**b.** Respiratory alkalosis
COPD _____	**c.** Metabolic acidosis
Pain _____	**d.** Metabolic alkalosis
Renal failure _____	
Fever _____	
Low potassium _____	
Drug overdose _____	

4. What acid-base disturbance do the following ABG values indicate? pH—7.33, P_aO_2—75, P_aCO_2—30, HCO_3^-—18?

Is compensation present?

5. Indicate whether the value represents acidosis, alkalosis, or a normal status:

pH	Acidosis	Alkalosis	Normal
a. 7.38			
b. 7.50			
c. 7.40			
d. 7.28			
e. 6.92			
f. 7.80			
g. 7.31			
h. 7.42			

6. Indicate whether the level of ventilation is increased (hyperventilation), decreased (hypoventilation), or normal:

pH	P_aCO_2	Hypo-ventilation	Hyper-ventilation	Normal
a. 7.02	70			
b. 7.35	50			
c. 7.50	26			
d. 7.38	38			
e. 7.22	28			
f. 7.31	58			

7. Indicate whether the value is normal, or whether it represents respiratory acidosis or respiratory alkalosis:

pH	P_aCO_2	Normal	Respiratory acidosis	Respiratory alkalosis
a. 7.22	71	_____	_____	_____
b. 7.39	42	_____	_____	_____
c. 7.50	30	_____	_____	_____
d. 7.30	50	_____	_____	_____
e. 7.16	80	_____	_____	_____
f. 7.56	26	_____	_____	_____
g. 7.40	39	_____	_____	_____

8. Indicate whether the value is normal, or whether it represents metabolic acidosis or metabolic alkalosis:

pH	HCO_3^-	Normal	Metabolic acidosis	Metabolic alkalosis
a. 7.28	18	_____	_____	_____
b. 7.36	24	_____	_____	_____
c. 7.10	19	_____	_____	_____
d. 7.48	31	_____	_____	_____
e. 7.48	24	_____	_____	_____
f. 7.51	13	_____	_____	_____

9. In the following exercise, indicate:
The nature of the acid-base disturbance.
Whether compensation is present.
Whether compensation is renal or pulmonary.

pH	P_aCO_2	HCO_3^-	Nature of disturbance	Compensation present? Yes	No	If yes, Renal	Pulmonary
a. 7.28	63	25	____	____	____	____	____
b. 7.20	40	14	____	____	____	____	____
c. 7.52	40	35	____	____	____	____	____
d. 7.56	23	26	____	____	____	____	____

RESPIRATORY PROBLEMS

e. 7.48	30	31	___ ___ ___ ___ ___
f. 7.16	82	32	___ ___ ___ ___ ___
g. 7.36	68	35	___ ___ ___ ___ ___
h. 7.40	40	26	___ ___ ___ ___ ___

ANSWERS

1. Oxygenation, ventilation, acid-base balance.

2. Respiratory acidosis.

3. Diabetes **c**.

   Vomiting **d**.

   COPD **a**.

   Pain **b**.

   Renal failure **c**.

   Fever **b**.

   Low potassium **d**.

   Drug overdose **a**.

4. Metabolic acidosis. Yes, respiratory.

5. **a.** Normal.
   b. Alkalosis.
   c. Normal.
   d. Acidosis.
   e. Acidosis.
   f. Alkalosis.
   g. Acidosis.
   h. Normal.

6. **a.** Hypoventilation.
   b. Hypoventilation.
   c. Hyperventilation.
   d. Normal.
   e. Hyperventilation.
   f. Hypoventilation.

7. **a.** Respiratory acidosis.
   b. Normal.
   c. Respiratory alkalosis.
   d. Respiratory acidosis.
   e. Respiratory acidosis.
   f. Respiratory alkalosis.
   g. Normal.

8. a. Metabolic acidosis.
   b. Normal.
   c. Metabolic acidosis.
   d. Metabolic alkalosis.
   e. Alkalosis, not metabolic.
   f. Alkalosis, not metabolic; there is metabolic compensation.

9. a. Respiratory acidosis; no compensation.
   b. Metabolic acidosis; no compensation.
   c. Metabolic alkalosis; no compensation.
   d. Respiratory alkalosis; no compensation.
   e. Metabolic and respiratory alkalosis; no compensation.
   f. Respiratory acidosis; incomplete pulmonary compensation.
   g. Respiratory acidosis; complete pulmonary compensation.
   h. Normal.

CHAPTER

5

Chronic Obstructive Pulmonary Disease

OBJECTIVES

After completing this chapter, you will be able to:

1. Identify the physiologic changes that occur in COPD

2. List 10 signs and symptoms of COPD

3. List four nursing diagnoses in the management of COPD

4. Specify four elements in a teaching program for patients with COPD.

A. Introduction

1. Incidence

COPD is rapidly becoming one of the most significant health problems in this country. It is a major cause of death (the fatalities are actually higher than statistics indicate because people with COPD often succumb to heart failure or pneumonia secondary to COPD). COPD is most prevalent among men over 45 years of age who live in urban areas, but this is changing with the increase in women smokers. A smoker is 14 times more likely than a nonsmoker to die of COPD. Although there is little public awareness of COPD, it has significant social and economic consequences.

2. Definitions

a. Emphysema. This is a progressive, degenerative condition caused by damage to the alveolar septa and bronchiolar collapse. Destruction of the alveolar walls and connective tissue produces large alveolar sacs and loss of elastic recoil; this results in expiratory air flow obstruction because the lungs can no longer empty efficiently. Early bronchiolar collapse leads to increased airway resistance, and blebs and bullae often develop.

b. Chronic bronchitis. Bronchitis, an inflammation of the mucosal lining of the tracheobronchial tree, is usually caused by smoke or other inhaled irritants and infections. This inflammatory reaction leads to edema of the mucosa, hypertrophy of the bronchial mucous glands, increased mucus production, ciliary dysfunction, and consequently air flow obstruction. Bronchitis is defined as chronic if the cough and expectoration last at least 3 months a year for 2 consecutive years. Chronic bronchitis is also characterized by increased airway resistance on exhalation and may occur together with emphysema.

c. Asthma. This is characterized by sudden bronchospasm with contraction of the smooth muscles in the bronchioles, resulting in airway narrowing. There is also swelling of the mucosa with increased production of thick, tenacious mucus.

Asthma may or may not be associated with allergies and can occur with emphysema and bronchitis. In the early stages, asthma is intermittent and reversible with little lung impairment between attacks.

d. COPD. Occurring as the culmination or combination of bronchitis, asthma, and emphysema, COPD is a progressive, irreversible degenerative process (see Figure 5-1). The patient may have had an asthmatic or bronchitic condition at the outset, but it progresses to the point where it differs from the original disease entirely. Emphysematous changes are quite common in COPD, but severe cases may also lead to right heart failure (cor pulmonale caused by pulmonary vascular disease).

B. Pathophysiology

The increased work of breathing in COPD is attributable to several factors. Hyperinflation of the alveoli results in an increased functional residual capacity, which decreases the efficiency of alveolar air exchange. Thus, breathing requires

Figure 5-1 *The degenerative process in COPD*

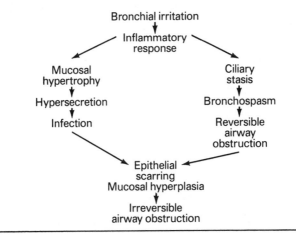

more work in order to achieve adequate ventilation. Destruction of the alveoli in COPD means less surface area for gas exchange. Since less alveolar gas is being exchanged with blood, there is more dead space (wasted) ventilation. This, too, means more work in breathing to provide adequate ventilation.

COPD also causes an uneven distribution of ventilation, creating hypoventilated areas in relation to blood flow. Unoxygenated venous blood therefore enters the bloodstream, leading to hypoxemia. This, in turn, increases the work load of both the heart and lungs.

The physiologic changes in the lung due to COPD cause $\dot{V}/\dot{Q}$ mismatching, hypoxemia, carbon dioxide retention, and acid-base disturbances. The disease progresses through the stages listed in Table 5-1, but not all patients develop hypoxemia and/or hypercapnia (increased P_aCO_2). It depends on the pathologic changes within the lungs and the progression of the disease. Because the heart must work harder to pump oxygenated blood to the tissues, it will eventually fail, and right heart failure (RHF) — cor pulmonale — will ensue.

C. Etiology

1. Smoking

This is the most important precipitating cause of COPD in the United States today. Not all smokers will develop COPD,

TABLE 5-1

STAGES IN SEVERITY OF EMPHYSEMA

Asymptomatic
Ventilatory deficit
Hypoxemia
Hypercapnia
Emphysematous heart disease (cor pulmonale)
    Compensated right heart failure (RVF)
    Uncompensated left heart failure (LVF)

but their chance of doing so far exceeds that of nonsmokers; a smoker with asthma will probably have more frequent and severe attacks.

2. Air pollution and occupation

Pollution and smog increase airway inflammation and bronchospasm, thereby worsening dyspnea. Irritating fumes and dust will aggravate COPD. Certain occupations that expose people to particulate matter or chemical irritants have been implicated as precipitating factors, but these are less significant than cigarette smoking.

3. Infections

Respiratory infections by themselves do not cause COPD, but recurrent infections that produce permanent lung damage may lead to it. Those with COPD are more susceptible to lung infections.

4. Heredity

One type of emphysema, due to an inherited deficiency of alpha$_1$-antitrypsin (a serum protein that inhibits the activity of elastase — an enzyme that breaks down elastic tissue), occurs in both men and women around 30 to 40 years of age, but it accounts for fewer than 4 percent of all cases.

5. Aging

COPD is more prevalent among older people, partly because of the increased period of time that cigarette smokers have been smoking.

6. Allergy

Since allergies play a significant role in the development of asthma, skin testing and hyposensitization are important.

D. Clinical picture and nursing assessment

1. Signs and symptoms

The following physical findings are common in patients with COPD, but the nature and severity of the illness do not depend on the number or type of findings present. In the area of the head there may be papilledema (increased P_aCO_2 causes vasodilation), cyanosis (central), pursed lip breathing, headaches, and diaphoresis.

About the chest and neck may be found an increased A-P diameter, a decreased diaphragmatic excursion (flattened), use of accessory muscles for breathing, hyperexpanded and rigid rib cage, hyperresonance (on percussion), breath sounds diminished with prolonged expiration, wheezes and rhonchi, rales (early inspiration), shortness of breath, neck vein distention, increased coughing and sputum production, tachycardia, and tachypnea.

In the abdominal area there may be evidence of increased development of abdominal musculature and an enlarged liver (if cor pulmonale is present).

The hands and nails may show clubbing, cyanosis (a late sign), and asterixis (liver flap due to increased P_aCO_2).

Neurologic signs and symptoms include judgment and personality change, restlessness, apprehension, anxiety, lethargy, drowsiness, confusion, coma (if severe or end-stage), sleeping difficulties, and nightmares.

2. Pulmonary function studies

These can often identify airway obstruction not detectable by physical examination or chest X-ray. However, these studies do not diagnose specific types of airway obstruction and are not an early diagnostic tool.

The patient with COPD would have decreased forced expiratory volume ($\downarrow$FEV), decreased vital capacity ($\downarrow$VC), decreased maximum midexpiratory flow rate ($\downarrow$MMEFR), increased functional residual capacity ($\uparrow$FRC), and normal or increased total lung capacity (N or $\uparrow$TLC) from air trapping (see Table 1-1).

3. Chest X-ray

On X-ray the chest will appear hyperradiolucent with decreased vascular markings. The diaphragm may be low and flat. A lateral view will show increased space between the hilus and the sternum. The heart may be small and vertical or enlarged (due to cor pulmonale).

4. ABGs

These can help to determine physiologic changes in those with severe COPD by identifying the presence and degree of hypoxemia, acidosis, hypercapnia, and renal compensation. Table 5-2 summarizes the ABG findings you'd be likely to encounter in acute and chronic advanced disease.

5. Other lab studies

The following studies may also help to identify the problem and its degree:
- Hematologic — polycythemia and eosinophilia
- Chemistries — nonspecific
- Sputum culture — secondary bacterial infections with either gram-negative or gram-positive organisms may occur; *Diplococcus pneumoniae* and *Haemophilus influenzae* are often found.

E. Complications of COPD

The following common complications are what we (as nurses) often see and care for in the acute care setting:

1. Cor pulmonale

Polycythemia (increased hematocrit and hemoglobin) develops to compensate for a low P_aO_2. This hypoxemia stimulates erythropoietin to increase RBC production. Thus, the heart must work harder to pump viscous blood around or to increase cardiac output in order to oxygenate

TABLE 5-2

ABG FINDINGS IN ACUTE AND CHRONIC ADVANCED COPD

ABG	Acute	Chronic with compensation
pH	↓	Normal
P_aCO_2	↑	↑
P_aO_2	↓	↓
HCO_3^-	Normal	↑

the tissues. The increased work causes the right ventricle to hypertrophy. Since the large volume of blood pumped into the pulmonary circulation is not well handled, the result is hypertension and ultimately the backup of blood into the vena cava, causing neck vein distention, ankle edema, and liver engorgement.

2. Acute respiratory failure (ARF)

As $\dot{V}/\dot{Q}$ mismatching worsens, hypoxemia and/or hypercapnia develop. Generally, a P_aO_2 less than 50 mm Hg and a P_aCO_2 greater than 50 mm Hg define ARF.

3. Pneumonia

Bacterial infections are particularly hard for COPD patients to overcome, and so increased mucus production and retention often lead to consolidation and pneumonia. Pneumonia may produce ARF in these patients. The most common causative organisms are *H. influenzae* and *D. pneumoniae*.

4. CO₂ narcosis

When COPD patients have a chronically high blood CO_2 level, the respiratory chemoreceptor centers in the brain are bombarded with messages to increase the level of ventilation in order to blow off the excess CO_2. But if the patient has an impaired ability to ventilate, this is not possible. The brain will soon become insensitive (or narcotized) to the CO_2 level as its stimulus to breathe, and then a hypoxic drive will stimulate respirations. This is why COPD patients usually receive only low-flow oxygen when treated for hypoxia (oxygenation

Figure 5-2   *Action of sympathomimetics and methylxanthines in COPD*

Stimulation by sympathomimetics		Inhibition by methylxanthines	
↓		↓	
(adenylate cyclase)	Cyclic AMP	(phosphodiesterase)	AMP
	↓		
	bronchodilation		

needs to be improved, but not to the point of removing the hypoxic drive).

5. Ulcers

There is a higher incidence of peptic ulcer disease among COPD patients, but the mechanism is not clear.

F. Treatment

Treatment should consist of the four following aspects:

1. Management of hypoxemia

Since hypoxia is potentially lethal, it must be reversed. However, too much inhaled oxygen will raise the P_aO_2 so high that the hypoxic drive — the patient's stimulus to breathe — will be destroyed and the patient may experience respiratory depression. Thus, low-flow oxygen delivery is recommended by means of a Venturi mask, nasal cannula, or simple or aerosol mask. It may be administered continuously or used only at night, depending on the degree of hypoxemia and the subsequent right ventricular hypertrophy. Intermittent oxygen therapy should not be used in managing COPD.

2. Airway management

The airway must be opened as wide as possible and kept free of obstruction (secretions) by means of bronchodilator therapy, bronchial hygiene, and humidification.

a. Bronchodilator therapy. Two types of drugs are used for bronchodilation — sympathomimetics and methylxanthines. Figure 5-2 shows how they act. They are often used together in order to enhance the potency and minimize the side effects of each. Sympathomimetics include isoproterenol hydrochloride (Isoprel), metaproterenol (Alupent, Metaprel), isoetharine (Bronkosol), epinephrine, terbutaline (Brethine, Bricanyl), and albuterol (Ventolin, Proventil). Examples of xanthines are theophylline (Elixophyllin, Theo-Dur, Constant T), aminophylline, and oxtriphylline (Choledyl).

Although steroids may be able to open the airways, they should be used only as a last resort and with extreme caution because of their side effects. How steroids work in this situation is not known, but it may be through their anti-inflammatory effect or they may have a direct bronchodilation effect on the airways.

b. Bronchial hygiene. Secretions can be mobilized by means of controlled effective breathing and chest physiotherapy (CPT), including postural drainage and suctioning (see Chapters 13 and 14).

c. Humidification. Since systemic humidification is preferable, you should encourage the patient to drink about eight glasses of fluid a day. Otherwise, aerosol nebulizers, face tents, and ultrasonic nebulizers can be used to deliver moisture to the respiratory tract. Remember that whenever oxygen or compressed air is administered (except in emergencies), some source of humidity should also be applied to counteract the dry, irritating effects of those gases and to help liquefy the secretions. Expectorants such as acetylcysteine (Mucomyst) can be used, but they are generally not as effective in loosening secretions.

3. Antibiotic therapy

Infection is the most common cause of acute illness in COPD patients. Its early signs include increased amounts of sputum, increased thickness of sputum, changes in sputum color and odor, increased frequency of coughing, increased shortness of breath, increased difficulty raising sputum, and a rise in temperature.

Broad-spectrum antibiotics such as ampicillin or tetracycline are used to treat these early signs. Typical causative organisms are *H. influenzae* and *D. pneumoniae*. If the organism is resistant to the antibiotic used, the patient will be switched to another according to the results of sputum culture and sensitivity tests.

4. Teaching the patient to cope

It may be difficult to speak with the patient because of his anxiety over his inability to breathe. This anxiety can best be alleviated by teaching the patient how to cope with his disorder. This can be accomplished by setting realistic goals for him, listening carefully to what he has to say, and including his family in various activities and decisions. Most of all, the patient needs a sense of hope and he needs to be encouraged whenever possible. A teaching program should include a discussion of the following: the disease process, effective breathing and coughing, signs and prevention of infection, controlling the environment, bronchial hygiene, diet, medication, exercise conditioning, and relaxation techniques.

Since living with COPD is a lifelong matter, these patients need whatever type of education and exercise conditioning that will help them overcome feelings of helplessness and hopelessness. A pulmonary rehabilitation program is beneficial in helping them cope.

G. Nursing diagnosis and potential patient problems

Once a patient assessment has been made, the nursing diagnosis that broadly applies to COPD patients includes:

- Impaired gas exchange related to $\dot{V}/\dot{Q}$ inequality
- Ineffective airway clearance because of bronchoconstriction, increased mucus production, and ineffective cough
- Ineffective breathing pattern related to shortness of breath, mucus, bronchoconstriction, and airway irritants
- Deficit in self-care related to fatigue secondary to increased work of breathing and poor ventilation and oxygenation
- Reduction in exercise tolerance due to lowered energy level, hypoxemia, and ineffective breathing patterns
- Disturbance in body image and self-esteem stemming from less socialization, anxiety, depression, lower activity level, or the inability to work
- Potential for noncompliance with recommended care procedures at home.

QUIZ

1. Which of the following physiologic changes occur as a result of COPD?
   a. $\dot{V}/\dot{Q}$ mismatching
   b. Hypoxemia
   c. Carbon dioxide retention
   d. Increased pulmonary blood flow
   e. Acid-base disturbances

2. List six etiologic factors in the development of COPD:

3. List 10 assessment findings that may be present in the COPD patient:

4. List five complications that may develop in the COPD patient:

5. The two classes of bronchodilators are
_____ and _____.

6. List four elements in a COPD teaching program:

7. List two nursing diagnoses for the COPD patient:

ANSWERS

1. **a, b, c, e.**

2. Smoking, air pollution and occupation, age, heredity, infection, allergy.

3. Restlessness, anxiety, papilledema, accessory muscle use, rigid rib cage, pursed lip breathing, shortness of breath, mucus production, coma, confusion, cyanosis, headaches, clubbing, diaphoresis, neck vein distention, personality change, tachycardia, tachypnea, diminished breath sounds, asterixis, prolonged expiration.

4. Cor pulmonale, acute respiratory failure, pneumonia, CO_2 narcosis, ulcers.

5. Sympathomimetics; methylxanthines.

6. Disease process, relaxation technique, effective breathing and coughing, signs and prevention of infection, controlling the environment, bronchial hygiene, diet, medications, exercise conditioning.

7. Reduction in exercise tolerance, change in body image.

6

Restrictive
Lung Disease

OBJECTIVES

After completing this chapter, you will be able to:

1. *Identify what pulmonary function values are affected in restrictive lung disease*

2. *List two types of restrictive disorders and the main characteristics of each*

3. *List the nursing assessment findings for these two disorders.*

A. Definition

A restrictive lung disease is one in which the individual's ability to inhale is impaired. Lung compliance is diminished because of pathophysiology and so the patient must work harder to breathe. In restrictive disease, the total lung capacity (TLC) is reduced and vital capacity (VC) is less than predicted (see Figure 1-2). The TLC may reflect a decrease in inspiratory reserve volume (IRV), tidal volume (V_T), expiratory reserve volume (ERV), and residual volume (RV) (as in atelectasis); a decrease in VC (IRV+V_T+ERV) with little involvement of residual volume (as in the surgical patient); or a decrease in functional residual capacity (ERV+RV) with variable involvement of IRV and V_T (as in adult respiratory distress syndrome [ARDS]).

B. Types

1. Atelectasis

There are two forms of this alveolar collapse: diffuse or patchy atelectasis, which occurs throughout the lung and cannot be seen on chest X-ray, and segmental or lobar atelectasis (more common), which involves only a region of the lung and can be seen on chest X-ray. Atelectasis may be caused by pleural fluid, pneumothorax, thoracic lesions, or (most often) retained secretions. It precedes hypostatic pneumonia, a common complication of acutely ill patients. The best treatment for retained secretions is aggressive respiratory therapy (see Chapter 14).

2. Central nervous system depression

Anything that depresses the brain's respiratory center will affect respiration by decreasing TLC — for example, drugs, anesthesia, and unconsciousness. So, a very real problem for any unconscious patient is the possible development of a restrictive lung condition with a potential for producing hypoxemia, hypercapnia, acidosis, atelectasis, pneumonia, obstruction, and aspiration. Here again, respiratory therapy is needed.

3. Neuromuscular disease

Any disease that affects the bellows mechanism of the lung by weakening its ventilatory capacity will generally cause a decline in all lung volumes. Such diseases include Guillain-Barré syndrome, myasthenia gravis, polio, spinal cord injury, muscular dystrophy, and tetanus.

Most of the lung conditions caused by these disorders are potentially reversible since the patients have essentially normal lungs. If these patients can be supported, by means of respiratory care, through episodes of acute ventilatory insufficiency, they can recover completely. The major nursing goals are to maintain airway patency and to monitor ventilatory capacity with supportive care.

4. The postoperative patient

Patients undergoing abdominal and thoracic surgery can develop a restrictive lung disorder due to decreased VC. The physiologic stress and pain of the surgical procedure make it extremely difficult for the patient to ventilate and clear his lungs. The resulting breathing problems will be due to poor ventilatory reserve and the resulting hypoxemia will be due to venous admixture; these conditions can readily be corrected with ventilator support and oxygen therapy.

The degree of restrictive disease in each surgical patient is fairly predictable; it is greatest in those undergoing upper abdominal surgery with abnormal pulmonary function studies, in those who have smoked, and in those over 60 years of age.

A patient's VC generally decreases between 12 and 18 hours after surgery, not immediately postoperatively. This has important implications for nursing care. You should make a thorough *preoperative* evaluation to identify those who are at high risk of developing postoperative pulmonary complications and also provide the supportive care necessary to maintain clear lungs.

5. Pulmonary fibrosis

This term implies the presence of an excessive amount of connective tissue in the lungs. *Localized* fibrosis (affecting a small section of one lung) is usually caused by tissue necrosis following pneumonitis, pulmonary abscess, tuberculosis, or the aspiration of vomitus. *Generalized* fibrosis (the diffuse involvement of both lungs) follows either a widespread pulmonary infection or the inhalation of irritating dust or noxious fumes (see Chapter 7). Because diffuse interstitial fibrosis is produced by an allergic or inflammatory process involving the lung parenchyma, it will vary in extent. The inhalation of organic dust antigens may cause bronchiolar and alveolar reactions that later lead to fibrotic changes.

6. Pulmonary consolidation

Although pneumonias are thought to be restrictive disorders, they will be discussed in Chapter 9, on infections.

7. ARDS

This is also viewed as a restrictive disorder but will be discussed in Chapter 12.

C. Assessment

In assessing patients with restrictive lung disease, look for the following:

1. Atelectasis

This may be identified by decreased expansion of the affected area, decreased or absent tactile or vocal fremitus, dull sound to percussion, decreased or absent breath sounds, bronchophony or whispered pectoriloquy (if secretion-related), rales (if secretion-related), dyspnea, and elevated temperature.

2. Central nervous system depression

The following characteristics may be noted: bradypnea or apnea, decreased bilateral lung expansion, diminished breath sounds, and signs of hypoxia.

3. Neuromuscular disease

This disease tends to produce ineffective lung excursion, substernal retractions, dyspnea, anxiety, and shallow, rapid respirations.

4. Postoperative patient

In this patient you may observe diminished or absent breath sounds, ineffective, weak cough, inability to take deep breaths (decreased VC), splinting above or over the incision, and slight temperature elevation.

5. Pulmonary fibrosis

The two types may be distinguished as follows: *Localized* fibrosis produces dyspnea on exertion, usually in upper lobes (if due to TB), restricted movement on affected side, dull or flat percussion note, increased tactile fremitus, diminished bronchovesicular breath sounds, rales, and deviation of the trachea t˜ the affected side.

Generalized or *diffuse* fibrosis causes dyspnea on exertion, decreased percussion note, increased tactile fremitus, bronchovesicular breath sounds, coarse inspiratory rales, and deviation of the trachea to the more affected side.

D. Treatment

The goal is to improve ventilation either by facilitating the mechanics of breathing (by breathing techniques, incentive spirometry, and mechanical ventilation) or by keeping the airway patent (by chest physiotherapy, including adequate postural drainage, and therapeutic bronchoscopy if indicated, coughing and effective suctioning, and antibiotic therapy).

E. Nursing goals

These include adequate ventilatory effort, maintenance of adequate airway patency and bronchial hygiene, prevention of infection, getting the patient to cough and raise secretions, reduction of patient's and family's anxiety, and improved lung volumes and reduced dyspnea.

QUIZ

1. For the following pulmonary function tests, indicate whether each would be increased, normal, or decreased in restrictive disorders.

　　a. TLC _____

　　b. VC _____

2. Match the restrictive disorder with the appropriate description:

Atelectasis _____

Neuromuscular disorder _____

Pulmonary fibrosis _____

Postoperative patient _____

a. Excessive connective tissue in the lungs
b. Stress and pain result in decreased VC
c. Alveolar collapse
d. Diseases that affect bellows mechanism

3. Match assessment findings with the restrictive disorders:

Atelectasis _____

Neuromuscular disorder _____

Pulmonary fibrosis _____

Postoperative patient _____

a. Rales
b. Decreased tactile fremitus or breath sounds
c. Splinting above or over the incision
d. Weakened musculature

ANSWERS

1. a. Decreased.
　　b. Decreased.

2. Atelectasis **c.**
　　Neuromuscular disorder **d.**
　　Pulmonary fibrosis **a.**
　　Postoperative patient **b.**

3. Atelectasis **b.**
　　Neuromuscular disorder **d.**
　　Pulmonary fibrosis **a.**
　　Postoperative patient **c.**

CHAPTER

7

Occupational Lung Diseases

OBJECTIVES

After completing this chapter, you will be able to:

1. *List three occupational lung diseases and the job setting where each can be acquired*

2. *Assess a patient who is at high risk of developing an occupational lung disease*

3. *Instruct someone who is exposed to airborne particles or pollutants on the job about what preventive measures can be taken.*

A. Incidence

People develop occupational lung diseases because of exposure to airborne particles and pollutants in their places of work. Although all types of people are affected, occupational lung diseases are more common among those who work in industries that emit particulate matter in the course of mining or manufacturing. Some of these diseases are obviously job-related (i.e., asbestosis affects asbestos workers), but many people simply develop chronic bronchitis, asthma, emphysema, or cancer at above-average levels in the course of their work. These nonspecific occupational diseases may actually affect more people than the job-specific diseases.

Most occupational lung diseases worsen with continued exposure—sometimes slowly and sometimes rapidly. The damage can be reversed only if stopped in the early stages. Usually, however, treatment can only slow down the relentless course. Patients with these diseases typically spend the rest of their lives wheezing, coughing, having chest pain, and often dying prematurely.

There are no statistics on the exact number of people who have occupational lung diseases, but the Department of Health and Human Services estimates that about 400,000 people develop a job-related disease every year. The department also estimates that about 100,000 deaths each year are due to occupational diseases, half of which are respiratory in nature. In addition, the World Health Organization estimates that 75 percent of all human cancers are either caused or aggravated by environmental factors, including diet, living habits, stress, chemicals, and smoking.

It is estimated that about $5 billion a year is paid out in workers' compensation for job-related illnesses and injuries. Beyond these statistics, however, is the human suffering— physical and emotional—including economic loss, family strains, and medical costs.

B. Diagnosis

It is not necessarily easy to recognize the relationship between the job and the particular disease because many occupational diseases develop very slowly over a number of years, so that many patients are not aware of becoming ill. Also, at the beginning of a disease, the patient may simply experience some coughing, shortness of breath, and colds. Nothing dramatic happens to motivate the individual to seek medical help. Meanwhile, his lungs are becoming increasingly inflamed, obstructed, stiffened, or overdistended.

Even if the individual consults a health professional, the disease may still not be recognized because his clinical picture resembles the one caused by heavy smoking, air pollution, or repeated infections. As a nurse, you should take a thorough working/occupational history of each patient you evaluate. Ask the patient about the various types of jobs he has had since he first started working. Possibly the 6-month period he spent working with asbestos 20 years ago is now causing his breathing problem.

Remember that a history of smoking will often present the same clinical picture as an occupational lung disease, but that you need to learn about the patient's various jobs as well because the combined effects of cigarette smoke and occupational dusts, gases, fumes, and vapors are extremely severe. Smokers get occupational lung diseases more often than do nonsmokers, and they die sooner from the effects of their disease. The risk of COPD, cancer, and heart disease is multiplied in the person who smokes and also works in a potentially hazardous environment.

C. Major occupational lung diseases

There are two major groups of occupational lung diseases: the *pneumoconioses*, caused by dust in the lungs, and the *hypersensitivity diseases*, caused by the lungs' overreaction to airborne pollutants (this group also includes occupational asthma and allergic alveolitis). Other common occupational lung diseases include byssinosis, industrial bronchitis, occupational lung cancers, and diseases caused by irritant gases.

Table 7-1 summarizes the various occupational diseases, the job settings where each may develop, a typical history leading to the development, the common signs and symptoms, and some preventive measures that can be taken.

TABLE 7-1

OCCUPATIONAL LUNG DISEASES

Disorder	Susceptible workers and industries	History
Pneumoconioses		
Silicosis	Foundry workers, pottery makers; glass, tile, and brick cutters Stone masons, sand-blasters Miners (lead, coal, gold, silver, copper, etc.)	Exposure to silica dust *Chronic:* 10-20 years' exposure to low concentrations (most common form) *Complicated:* fibrosis develops from chronic exposure *Acute:* intense exposure over short time (weeks to months). Progresses rapidly, leading to disability and death within 5 years
Black lung disease (coal workers' pneumoconiosis [CWP])	Coal miners (10-20% of all coal miners affected)	More prevalent among miners of anthracite (rather than bituminous) coal *Simple CWP:* exists without other lung conditions *Complicated CWP:* fibrosis develops
Asbestosis	Mining, milling, tile-making, manufacturing (insulating materials, paint, cement, clutch and brake linings, etc.) Heating and insulation workers, demolition workers, electricians, clothing ironers, construction workers, shipbuilders, decorators, painters	Exposure to asbestos products whether at place of work or other environment Fibrosis develops usually after 10-20 years' exposure Lung cancer associated with all types of asbestos exposure (20-30% of deaths among asbestos workers is due to lung cancer) Greatest incidence among heavy smokers
Mixed dust pneumoconioses	Foundry, steel, iron workers	Exposure to various dusts or fumes by changing jobs

Signs and symptoms	Prevention and treatment
Chronic: breathlessness during exercise, cough and sputum *Complicated:* breathlessness, weakness, chest pain, cough, sputum *Acute:* dyspnea, weight loss, fever, coughing	Dust control Improved ventilation Wetting-down of mines Use of respirator
Simple CWP: none *Complicated CWP:* dyspnea, heart failure, productive cough, wheezing	Dust control
Cough, sputum, weight loss, wheezing or rales, increased shortness of breath	Tighter controls on use of asbestos Shower and change clothing at job site
Same as for each component type of dust Severity of fibrosis related to amount of silica exposure	

TABLE 7-1 (continued)

Disorder	Susceptible workers and industries	History
Hypersensitivity diseases		
Occupational asthma	Antigen found in the workplace (e.g., dog hair for kennel workers) Detergent enzymes, platinum salts, cereals and grains, certain wood dusts, chemicals used in polyurethane products, some pesticides	10% of population have inherited tendency toward allergies. They are inclined to develop occupational asthma (usually in less than 5 years)
Allergic alveolitis	Occupational exposure to moldy hay (farmers' lung), moldy sugarcane, barley, maple bark, cork, animal hair, bird feathers and droppings, mushroom compost, coffee beans, paprika, certain chemicals (especially isocyanate chemicals) Note: fungus spores growing in the antigen may be the real cause of the disease	Symptoms begin hours after exposure to offending dust and may last 10 days If dust exposure is infrequent or concentration is low, symptoms may not be recognized by worker Chronic alveolitis may lead to irreversible fibrosis
Byssinosis (brown lung)	Textile industry Flax and hemp industries Cotton workers	Called "Monday fever" since symptoms appear on Monday (or first day back to work after vacation or days off). They disappear on subsequent work days Most prevalent among workers involved in early stages of processing Onset may develop after a few months or many years of exposure

Signs and symptoms	Prevention and treatment
Wheezing, tenacious sputum Dyspnea, "tight chest," rhinor- rhea, sneezing	Avoid occupation with known antigen Treat with bronchodilators, antihis- tamines, and steroids
Fatigue Shortness of breath Dry cough Fever, chills	Separate worker from antigen Treat with steroids and other drugs. Patient may take 6 weeks to re- cover or there may be residual lung damage
Tight feeling in chest, cough, dyspnea Initially symptoms appear only on Monday; later on, they per- sist throughout the week. Eventually worker gets no re- lief and chronic bronchitis and emphysema develop (with dyspnea, persistent produc- tive cough, and chest pain)	Dust control Pretreat bales of cotton by washing with steam Pick cotton by hand (fewer causa- tive agents are thereby picked) Stop smoking

TABLE 7-1 (continued)

Disorder	Susceptible workers and industries	History
Industrial bronchitis	A controversial term: many feel that bronchitis due mainly to workplace pollutants should be called "industrial bronchitis." Others feel it is not clear the bronchitis is mainly occupational in origin (especially since it is aggravated by cigarette smoking)	Exposure to an irritant—air pollution, cigarette smoke, dust, irritant gases, vapors—in the workplace
Occupational lung cancer	Cigarette smoking is single most important cause; 70-90% of all cancers are due in part to environmental factors (including occupational exposure and air pollution) Lung cancer rates above average in occupations that handle: arsenic, bis-chloromethyl ether, coal tar, pitch volatiles, petroleum, mustard gas, coal carbonization products, chromates, asbestos, X-rays, radium, uranium, nickel, isopropyl oils Increased risk among chemists, painters, and printers	Lung cancer is more prevalent in industrialized and urban areas Symptoms seldom appear until the disease is well advanced
Irritant gases that cause lung disease		
Sulfur dioxide	Chemical plants Petroleum refineries Smelting (copper, lead, and zinc ore) Refrigeration industry Ice manufacturing Dried fruit industry Exposure to fuel combustion	Exposure results in susceptibility to lung infections and chronic lung disease

Signs and symptoms	Prevention and treatment
Same as chronic bronchitis Persistent cough and production of sputum	Change occupation Good ventilation in workplace No smoking in workplace
Dyspnea, productive cough	*Stop smoking* Carcinogenic substances in workplace should be controlled or replaced with safer materials Often not treatable because too advanced by the time it is diagnosed
Irritates respiratory tract; causes increased coughing, dry throat, burning feeling in upper respiratory tract Continued exposure may cause fatigue, loss of sense of smell, increased mucus production, and shortness of breath	The elderly, children, and those with lung or cardiac disorders should avoid exposure to high levels of SO_2 Proper ventilation Respirators for areas where gas level is above 5 ppm Protective clothing needed around liquid SO_2

TABLE 7-1 (continued)

Disorder	Susceptible workers and industries	History
Chlorine	Manufacturing (refrigerants, pesticides, synthetic rubber, plastics) Workers who handle chlorine for purifying drinking water, disinfecting swimming pools, and treating sewage	This is a heavy, greenish yellow gas with a pungent odor that warns of exposure. However, regular exposure may depress one's ability to detect it at low concentrations
Phosgene	Manufacturing (dyes, insecticides, pharmaceuticals) Firefighters	Sweet but unpleasant odor Chronic exposure may cause COPD
Ozone	Arc welding, aging liquor and wood Drying varnishes and ink	Bluish, pungent gas; helps produce smog
Nitrogen dioxide	Enters atmosphere as by-product of natural gas combustion, after explosions, in industries using nitric acid, and in motor vehicle emissions Manufacturing (rocket fuels, fertilizers, dyes, pharmaceuticals, chemicals) Jewelry-making, food bleaching, gas and electric arc welding, lithographing, electroplating, silo filling High concentrations in cigarette smoke	Has a reddish brown hue and is key component of smog Smoking is major contributor to respiratory disease; NO_2 goes deeply into lungs and can cause extensive damage before first symptoms appear
Ammonia	Manufacturing (fertilizers, explosives, dyes, plastics) Industries (refrigeration; petroleum refining; chemical, pharmaceutical, and leather tanning)	

Signs and symptoms	Prevention and treatment
Burning sensation felt in mucous membranes of eyes, nose, throat, and lungs Continued exposure causes chest pain, coughing, and sometimes vomiting May cause tracheal and bronchial edema and spasm	Respirators needed when level is above 1 ppm Full protective clothing needed during and shower after exposure to liquid form
Irritates upper respiratory tract Liquid form may cause burns Dizziness, chills, thirst, cough, thick sputum Continued exposure leads to pulmonary edema	Full face mask and air respirator needed when concentration is high Protective clothing needed when liquid is used (more than 0.1 ppm)
Coughing, choking, headaches, severe fatigue Effects aggravated during exercise After exposure ceases, pulmonary edema can develop	Use gas masks and full face goggles or respirators if concentration is above 0.1 ppm
Acute exposure to high concentrations can cause severe illness—even collapse and death It attacks tissues slowly, causing scarring and permanent lung disorders	Levels above 5 ppm are dangerous In confined areas where NO_2 can accumulate, goggles and respirators are necessary Proper ventilation needed Stop smoking
Intensely irritating to mucous membranes Produces headache, salivation, burning in throat, perspiration, nausea, vomiting, and pain below sternum	Proper ventilation Respirators needed if exposure is great Full protective clothing needed if liquid is being handled

D. Nursing goals

Nursing care of patients with occupational lung disease involves three aspects:

- Determining which patients are at high risk of developing an occupational disease by taking a thorough occupational history of all patients with generalized respiratory symptoms who are seen in a clinical setting (acute or nonacute)
- Educating those who are exposed to an environmental hazard of the risks of continued exposure, of ways to decrease its potential danger, and of the risks of cigarette smoking
- Providing acute care during an infectious episode and in advanced stages if the patient develops ARF or cor pulmonale.

QUIZ

1. Match the occupational lung disease with the category of worker who may develop it:

Coal miners _____   **a.** Byssinosis

Heating and insulation   **b.** Black lung
workers _____
                             c. Allergic alveolitis
Cotton workers _____
                             d. Asbestosis
Farmers who work with
moldy hay, etc. _____

2. In order to identify those who are at high risk of developing an occupational lung disease, it may be more important to take a thorough _____ _____ rather than a physical examination.

3. List three common signs that may be present in any patient with an occupational lung disease:

4. Of the following, which are the three most realistic preventive measures that people in environmentally hazardous workplaces should be taught?
  a. Stop smoking
  b. Change jobs
  c. Dust-control measures
  d. Proper ventilation or use of respirators
  e. Take off sick time regularly to reduce exposure

ANSWERS

  1. Coal miners **b.**
     Heating and insulation workers **d.**
     Cotton workers **a.**
     Farmers who work with moldy hay, etc. **c.**
  2. Occupational history.
  3. Wheezing, shortness of breath, coughing.
  4. a, c, d.

8

Pulmonary Vascular Disease

OBJECTIVES

After completing this chapter you will be able to:

1. *Identify patients who are at high risk of developing a pulmonary embolus and the assessment factors that indicate an embolus, and specify at least two approaches to treatment*

2. *Identify which patients are in pulmonary edema; list the possible causes; and specify the components of treatment*

3. *Define pulmonary hypertension; and list three causes and three signs and symptoms.*

A. Pulmonary embolism

One of the most common pulmonary complications seen in hospitalized patients, pulmonary embolism is defined as a partial or complete obstruction of one or both of the pulmonary arteries or their subdivisions. In most cases, it is caused by a clot that has become dislodged from a deep vein in the leg. The bigger the clot, the greater the lung tissue damage, and the more critical the situation.

Proper diagnosis is the key to managing patients with pulmonary embolism. Most of the symptoms are nonspecific and could be attributed to any pulmonary ailment. The nurse plays an important role in identifying the high-risk patient and in trying to prevent pulmonary embolism.

1. Etiology or predisposing factors

Anyone with a condition that can lead to deep vein thrombosis (DVT) is at risk of developing pulmonary embolism (see Table 8-1).

2. Pathophysiology

Three factors predispose to clot formation (Virchow's triad):
- Hypercoagulability of the blood, which can occur during pregnancy or postoperatively; in those with a fever or certain malignancies; in those using oral contraceptives
- Venous injury due to trauma or disease which alters the integrity of the blood vessel walls
- Venous stasis which causes clots and their extension.

Two mechanisms cause thrombi to become dislodged or to fragment:
- Direct trauma, sudden muscle action, or changes in blood flow that alter intravascular pressures
- The natural mechanism of clot dissolution.

The pulmonary embolus causes an inadequate supply of blood to a wedge-shaped area of the lung, producing alveolar changes; the resultant $\dot{V}/\dot{Q}$ abnormality causes arterial hypoxemia. The reduced vascular bed in the lung may increase pulmonary vascular resistance. The pulmonary artery pressure then rises (pulmonary hypertension), producing a strain on the right ventricle and sometimes lead-

TABLE 8-1

RISK FACTORS FOR DEEP VEIN THROMBOSIS

Prolonged immobility	Trauma or fractures of lower extremities
Recent surgery	Certain tumors
Obesity	Oral contraceptives
Advanced age	Pre-existing lung or heart disease
Pregnancy and postpartum	

ing to heart failure. Two other events may be precipitated by a pulmonary embolus: pulmonary hemorrhage and pulmonary infarction.

3. Nursing assessment

The patient's symptoms and condition depend upon the size and location of the embolus. The onset of symptoms in some patients will be sudden, but in others the symptoms will be more subtle.

a. Signs and symptoms. These include pleuritic chest pain, dyspnea, cough, anxiety or apprehension, hemoptysis, syncope, swelling, pain, warmth and tenderness in leg (if there is thrombosis), and cyanosis and shock (in massive pulmonary embolus).

b. Assessment findings. You may note tachypnea, tachycardia, rales, loud P_2 (pulmonic second sound), S_3 gallop, elevated temperature, pleural friction rub, and decreased breath sounds.

c. Laboratory tests. These show elevated WBC and sedimentation rate, decreased P_aO_2, and decreased P_aCO_2 (hyperventilation).

d. ECG. This is consistent with right ventricular failure.

e. Perfusion lung scan. Absence of radioactivity indicates areas of diminished or absent blood flow.

f. Ventilation lung scan. When combined with perfusion lung scan, this can be helpful in making the diagnosis. Initially the ventilation lung scan will be normal.

g. Pulmonary angiography. A definitive diagnosis can be made by catheterizing the right side of the heart.

4. Treatment

The goal should be prevention through such measures as deep breathing, coughing, incentive spirometry, turning, active or passive range of motion exercises, elastic stockings, leg elevation, and minidose heparin. These should be initiated early in the high-risk patient.

After pulmonary embolus has been diagnosed, treatment modalities include heparin, followed by warfarin sodium (Coumadin), oxygen for hypoxemia, streptokinase (Kabikinase, Streptase) or urokinase (Abbokinase) to dissolve the clot in massive embolus or ascending thrombophlebitis, vasopressors and fluids for hypotension, and surgery (vena cava interruption, transvenous umbrella, vena cava plication, pulmonary embolectomy).

5. Nursing goals

It is important to identify patients at high risk, institute preventive measures if there is DVT, provide symptomatic and supportive care, reduce the patient's anxiety and fear, provide for a quiet, nonstimulating environment, and teach about the use of anticoagulants.

B. Pulmonary edema

Normally, the lungs are prevented from accumulating a great deal of water. However, in certain disease states, transudation of fluid into the interstitium and alveolar space due to increased capillary pressure results in pulmonary edema.

1. Causes

Although the most common cause is left heart failure, pulmonary edema can also be due to widespread capillary damage, which produces a form of severe respiratory failure. (Noncardiogenic pulmonary edema will be discussed in Chapter 12.)

2. Pathophysiology

Normal lung water is maintained by the balance between capillary pressure and plasma osmotic pressure and by the integrity of normal capillary wall permeability. A disturbance in either or both of these will result in the transudation of fluid from the capillaries into the interstitial tissues and alveoli. The end result is that oxygen is unable to transfer across the alveolar capillary membrane, thereby causing hypoxemia.

3. Assessment

To identify those who are at high risk of developing pulmonary edema, look for the following: tachycardia, increased or decreased blood pressure, slightly elevated temperature, dyspnea, cyanosis, distended neck veins, orthopnea, rales over both lung bases, S_3 heart sound, and other clinical signs of hypoxia.

4. Treatment

Patient management includes treating the underlying cause; administering oxygen therapy, diuretics, and digitalis (as ordered); use of 20 to 50 percent ethyl alcohol solution in IPPB to decrease foaming; and monitoring for arrhythmias.

5. Nursing goals

These include improving oxygenation, monitoring hypoxia, providing for patient comfort, maintaining airway patency, and evaluating effectiveness of care.

C. Pulmonary hypertension

This occurs when the pulmonary artery pressure is elevated (Table 8-2). Primary pulmonary hypertension (idiopathic) —which is rare—occurs most often in women between 20 and 40 years of age and is fatal within 3 to 4 years. Secondary

TABLE 8-2

DEFINITION OF PULMONARY HYPERTENSION

PAP—systolic	> 30 mm Hg
PAP—diastolic	> 15 mm Hg
PAP—mean	> 20 mm Hg

pulmonary hypertension—which is more common—results from existing cardiac or pulmonary disease; its prognosis depends upon the severity of the underlying disorder.

1. Causes

The most common cause of pulmonary hypertension in the United States is alveolar hypoventilation due to COPD; see Table 8-3 for others.

2. Pathophysiology

Normally, the pulmonary vascular bed has a low resistance to flow and compensates for increased blood volume by opening unused vessels. However, if the vascular bed is destroyed or obstructed, as in pulmonary hypertension, this ability is lost and the increased blood flow then increases the pulmonary artery pressure (PAP). As the PAP increases, the pulmonary vascular resistance (PVR) also increases. This in-

TABLE 8-3

CAUSES OF PULMONARY HYPERTENSION

Primary	Altered immune mechanisms associated with collagen diseases
Secondary	Hypoxemia due to:
	Alveolar hypoventilation
	Hypoxia
	COPD
	Sarcoidosis
	Diffuse interstitial pneumonia
	Malignant metastases
	Scleroderma
	Obesity
	Kyphoscoliosis
	Vascular obstruction
	Pulmonary embolus
	Vasculitis
	Widespread interstitial disease
	Primary cardiac disease
	Congenital (patent ductus, atrial septal defect [ASD], ventricular septal defect [VSD])
	Acquired (rheumatic valvular disease, mitral stenosis)

creased pressure load affects right ventricular function and results in decreased cardiac output and right ventricular failure (RVF).

Another cause of increased PVR is vasoconstriction. In the pulmonary vascular bed, generalized hypoxia (from any source) causes vasoconstriction, which increases PVR.

Increased PVR invariably causes intrapulmonary shunting, hypoxemia, respiratory alkalosis followed by acidosis, and decreased mixed venous oxygen tension. The pathophysiologic progression is summarized in Figure 8-1.

3. Assessment and clinical picture

Since pulmonary hypertension is potentially fatal, it is extremely important that you recognize both the condition and those who are at risk.

a. Signs and symptoms. These include increasing dyspnea on exertion (most common); chest pain (in 30 to 60 percent of those affected); weakness, fatigability, syncope; signs of right heart failure (RHF) (peripheral edema, ascites, neck vein

Figure 8-1 *Pathophysiologic progression of pulmonary hypertension*

Pulmonary disorders (pulmonary embolus, COPD, altitude, drugs, hypoventilation, interstitial diseases)

Anatomic changes in pulmonary blood vessels

Reduction of pulmonary vascular bed

Functional changes in the lungs

Hypoxemia   Hypercapnia   Acidosis

Pulmonary arteriolar vasoconstriction

Increased pulmonary vascular resistance

Pulmonary hypertension

Right ventricular hypertrophy

Cor pulmonale (RVF)

distention, hepatomegaly, rales); ECG showing right ventricular hypertrophy, right axis deviation, and tall peaked P waves in inferior leads; and decreased P_aO_2 (hypoxemia).

b. Cardiac catheterization. This will show elevated pulmonary artery pressure; elevated pulmonary capillary wedge pressure (PCWP) in atrial myxoma, mitral stenosis, or LVF; and normal PCWP in all other causes.

c. Pulmonary angiography. This will detect defects in pulmonary vasculature such as pulmonary emboli.

d. Pulmonary function tests. In obstructive diseases there will be increased RV and TLC and decreased flow rates; and in restrictive diseases, decreased TLC and VC.

4. Treatment

The major component is oxygen therapy to reduce the hypoxemia and the resulting pulmonary vascular resistance. For patients with RHF, treatment should also include fluid restriction, digitalis to improve cardiac functioning, and diuretics to decrease fluid accumulation. The underlying cause must be treated whenever possible.

5. Nursing goals

It is important to correct hypoxemia by means of oxygen administration; monitor ABGs for acidosis and hypoxemia; control RHF by means of daily weighing, recording patient's intake and output, and restricting food and fluid intake; monitor cardiac and hemodynamic status; and help the patient adjust to limitations (especially overexertion).

QUIZ

1. What single condition predisposes a person to develop a pulmonary embolus?

2. List two signs and symptoms and two assessment findings that may be present in the patient with a pulmonary embolus:

3. List two approaches to treatment:

4. The most common cause of pulmonary edema is

   _____

5. List three assessment findings in the patient with pulmonary edema:

6. The major goal in managing the patient with pulmonary edema is _____ .

7. In pulmonary hypertension, the pulmonary artery systolic pressure is greater than _____ .

8. The three overall causes of secondary pulmonary hypertension are:

9. List three signs and symptoms that may be present in the patient with pulmonary hypertension:

ANSWERS

1. Deep vein thrombosis.

2. Signs and symptoms: dyspnea, cough, anxiety, pleuritic chest pain, hemoptysis, syncope, swelling and pain in extremity, cyanosis.

   Assessment findings: tachypnea, tachycardia, rales, P_2 and S_3 heart sound, elevated temperature, decreased breath sounds, pleural friction rub.

3. Prevention, heparin, oxygen, streptokinase, vasopressors and fluids, surgery.

4. Left heart failure.

5. Tachycardia, distended neck veins, rales over both lung bases, S_3 heart sound, dyspnea, cyanosis.

6. Treat the underlying cause.

7. 30 mm Hg.

8. Alveolar hypoventilation, vascular obstruction, primary cardiac disease.

9. Dyspnea on exertion, chest pain, weakness, syncope, signs of right heart failure, ECG changes, decreased P_aO_2.

Lung Infections

OBJECTIVES

After completing this chapter, you will be able to:

1. *Identify three of the major hospital-acquired pneumonias and three assessment findings of each*

2. *Explain how a lung abscess develops and list five typical assessment findings in a patient with a lung abscess*

3. *Define empyema and list four typical assessment findings in a patient with an empyema*

4. *Name the causative organism in tuberculosis and the four drugs most commonly used for treatment.*

A. Classification

Pulmonary infections are a common cause of lung dysfunction. They are classified as both obstructive and restrictive because the secretions produced can cause obstruction and restrict expansion of the lungs, thereby dramatically decreasing lung volume.

B. Pneumonias*

1. Incidence

This is an inflammatory disease of the parenchyma of the lungs. It is ranked as the fifth leading cause of death in the United States; together with influenza, it accounts for more fatalities than any other infectious disease.

2. Classification and etiology

Pneumonia can be classified as either hospital- or community-acquired. If it was acquired in the community and the patient had been in relatively good health, the organism responsible is probably either *Diplococcus pneumoniae*, *Mycoplasma*, or a virus. If the patient is elderly or has been compromised by a debilitating disease, he may be affected by more dangerous organisms such as *Staphylococcus aureus* or the gram-negative bacilli.

Gram-negative aerobic bacilli are also primarily responsible for hospital-acquired (nosocomial) pneumonias. Hospitalized patients may contract pneumonia as a result of early colonization of the oropharynx, aspiration, aerosolization from contaminated respiratory equipment, or any invasive procedure that introduces pathogens into the bloodstream. Table 9-1 lists the common hospital-acquired pneumonias.

3. Nursing goals

For pneumonia, it is important to help identify the causative organism, administer appropriate and specific antimicrobial therapy and evaluate its effectiveness, remove secretions from the bronchi, provide symptomatic and supportive care, pre-

*The section on pneumonias was contributed by Sally Ryan, R.N.

vent complications, make the patient comfortable, and teach the patient and his family about prevention, complications, and what appropriate action to take.

C. Lung abscess

This is a localized, pus-filled necrotic lesion in the lung. It may occur as a result of the aspiration of vomitus or infected material from the upper airway; or it may be secondary to tumor obstruction, tuberculosis, pulmonary embolism, chest trauma, or necrotizing pneumonia (see Table 9-2). Lung abscess is characterized by the formation of a cavity, which may or may not communicate with a bronchus initially. Eventually, it becomes surrounded by a wall of fibrous tissue with only one or two points of communication with either the lumen of some bronchus or the pleural space. If the cavity connects with a bronchus, the purulent contents are removed continuously via the sputum. If it connects with the pleural space, an empyema forms. If both avenues of communication exist, a bronchopleural fistula develops.

1. Assessment

The onset of symptoms may be insidious or acute. Usually, there will be malaise and fever with or without pleuritic pain. Then, over the next few days, you will probably note the following: low-grade fever, cough with sputum, dyspnea, foul-smelling breath (from pus), blood-tinged, purulent drainage (from bronchial erosion), malaise, dullness to percussion, decreased breath sounds with occasional rales, pleural friction rub, egophony, anemia, and weight loss (if chronic).

2. Treatment

The following are recommended: antibiotic therapy (specific to organism) usually for four to six weeks, chest physiotherapy (CPT), including postural drainage, and surgical intervention (lobectomy) if medical therapy is not successful.

3. Nursing goals

In the case of a lung abscess, it is important to establish adequate drainage with CPT, assist in treating infection, offer

TABLE 9-1

COMMON HOSPITAL-ACQUIRED PNEUMONIAS

Type	Transmission
Pneumococcal—accounts for 90% of all bacterial pneumonia (*Diplococcus* [*Streptococcus*] *pneumoniae*—gram-positive capsulated bacterium)	Inhalation of droplets Close person-to-person contact
Staphylococcal (*Staphylococcus aureus*—gram-positive aerobic bacterium)	Inhalation or aspiration Bloodstream sometimes transports septic emboli to lungs
Influenza virus pneumonia (groups A through D virus; D causes most pneumonias)	Person-to-person contact (by inhaling virus in droplets from infected persons)
Pseudomonas pneumonia—most dreaded nosocomial type (*Pseudomonas aeruginosa*—gram-negative aerobic bacterium)	Inhalation of organism—often from contaminated nebulizer or ventilator and frequent suctioning Sometimes from wound infection at site of intravenous catheter—causing bacteremia
Acute aspiration pneumonia (due to caustic hydrochloric acid in gastric juices)	While under anesthesia, during a seizure, or in coma, patient may aspirate gastric juices

RESPIRATORY PROBLEMS

Clinical signs	Treatment
Abrupt onset; high fever with shaking chills Cough productive of "rusty" or green-ish material, pleural pain, decreased breath sounds, dullness over site, crepitations Bacteremia is common On X-ray: homogeneous consolidation of lung parenchyma, not involving an entire lobe Atelectasis is common	Penicillin Erythromycin (for those sensitive to penicillin)
Infants: abrupt onset with cyanosis, tachypnea, high fever Hospitalized patients with compro-mised immune defenses: insidious onset, fever, cough productive of purulent, blood-streaked material, rales, rhonchi, decreased breath sounds; mortality high Nonhospitalized persons: abrupt onset, cough productive of purulent yellow or brown material, pleural pain frequent Abscess cavities occur in 25-75% of patients Pleural effusion and empyema occur in 50% of patients	Susceptibility pattern must be done to choose appropriate agent (this bacterium is resistant to many anti-microbials)
1-2 days after onset of influenza: high fever; cough productive of frothy, bloody sputum; substernal chest pain; dyspnea; expiratory wheezing; moist rales On X-ray: diffuse bilateral broncho-pneumonia radiating from hilus	Will not respond to antimicrobials
Abrupt onset, fever, chills, bradycardia, severe dyspnea Cough productive of copious yellow or green sputum (sometimes blood-streaked) If pneumonia due to bacteremia, ecthyma gangrenosa develops together with circulatory collapse On X-ray: posterior segments of lower lobes most severely involved	Susceptibility testing required
On X-ray: bilateral air space consoli-dation Areas of lung affected depend on pa-tient's position when he aspirated; pulmonary edema-like signs present	Corticosteroids Antibiotics

TABLE 9-1 (continued)

Type	Transmission
Pneumocystis pneumonia (interstitial) (*Pneumocystis carinii*)	Probably by inhalation
E. coli pneumonia (*Escherichia coli*—gram-negative bacillus)	Inhalation of droplets Neonates may aspirate amniotic fluid during birth Can be secondary to bacteremia
Mycoplasmal pneumonia (*Mycoplasma pneumoniae*—a pleuropneumonia-like organism [PPLO]—neither virus nor bacterium)	Inhalation of droplets Contact with oral secretions from infected person

emotional support, and teach steps in prevention, follow-up, signs of recurrence, and appropriate actions.

D. Empyema

Empyema is a collection of infected pleural exudate found between the visceral and parietal pleurae. At first the pleural fluid is thin, but then it may progress to a fibropurulent stage, and finally enclose the lung within a thick, exudative membrane. Empyema is usually associated with an underlying pulmonary infection following thoracic surgery or a penetrating chest wound.

Clinical signs	Treatment
Infants: low-grade fever, restlessness, feeding problems, tachypnea, cyanosis, mild productive cough, crepitant rales on deep breathing; can be fatal within few days Older children, adults: abrupt onset with spiking fever, tachypnea, productive cough; can be fatal within a week On X-ray: diffuse changes; consolidation with focal area of atelectasis and emphysema	Pentamidine isethionate (Lomidine)* Trimethoprim-sulfamethoxazole (Bactrim, Septra)
Abrupt onset Chills, fever, pleural pain, dyspnea Cough productive of thick, yellow sputum Possibly rales at lung bases and decreased breath sounds On X-ray: patchy or confluent bronchopneumonia	Susceptibility testing required
Malaise, headache, fever, cough, substernal pain Sputum production gradually increases Moist rales common URI symptoms On X-ray: early stages show fine, reticular pattern indicative of interstitial disease followed by patchy air space consolidation; tends to be segmental	Tetracycline Erythromycin

*Available from Centers for Disease Control, Atlanta, GA 30333.

1. Assessment

The following might be found in a patient with empyema: elevated temperature, pleural pain, dyspnea, anorexia, weight loss, absent breath sounds, dullness to percussion, decreased vocal fremitus, and leukocytosis. The pleural exudate should be examined by pleural biopsy (needle aspiration).

2. Treatment

The following measures are appropriate forms of therapy: remove infected material; use selective antibiotic therapy; drain fluid by means of thoracocentesis, closed chest drainage,

TABLE 9-2

COMMON CAUSES OF LUNG ABSCESS

Type of abscess	*Cause*
Aspiration	Alcoholism
	Postanesthesia
	Coma
	Oral infection
	Food or foreign body in lung
	Laryngeal palsy
Malignant	Necrotic bronchial carcinoma secondary to bronchial obstruction and stasis of secretions
	Head and neck malignancies
Pulmonary embolus	Pulmonary infarction
	Septic emboli
Infection	Pneumonia
	Defective ciliary action
	Inefficient expectoration
	Infected cysts
	Necrotic lesions
	Subphrenic infections
	Open chest wounds

open rib resection to remove thickened pleura and pus and resect underlying tissue; use underwater-seal drainage until pus-filled space is gone as determined by chest X-ray.

3. Nursing goals

These are the same as those listed for lung abscess.

E. Tuberculosis

Tuberculosis is one of the leading causes of fever of unknown origin. It results from the inhalation of droplet nuclei containing *Mycobacterium tuberculosis*. These nuclei are emitted into the air by patients with active disease, especially when they cough. We now know that minimal exposure to someone with tuberculosis is unlikely to produce infection in most people; one must inhale contaminated air for many months before contracting the disease.

Most infections completely resolve before any symptoms appear. However, reactivation, or reinfection, tuberculosis may appear within 2 or 3 years. This is why conversion of the tuberculin reaction is a major indication for preventive chemotherapy. This type of tuberculosis generally develops in the upper portions of the lung, where there is more ventilation than perfusion—a favorable environment for the aerobic tubercle bacillus.

1. Assessment

The findings will vary, depending on the severity and involvement of the lung, but they include cough, fever, malaise, hemoptysis, positive tuberculin test, sputum positive for *Mycobacterium tuberculosis*, and X-rays showing areas of infiltration with one or more areas of cavitation.

2. Treatment

The principal treatment is effective chemotherapy. Patients are usually given two or more different drugs, depending on sensitivity, for several months until their X-ray shows a stable condition and their sputum cultures are negative. It is then recommended that they take the medication daily for an additional 12 months for maximum resolution of the infection and to prevent a relapse. Table 9-3 lists the drugs most commonly used for tuberculosis.

TABLE 9-3

CHEMOTHERAPY FOR TUBERCULOSIS

Drug	Daily dosage	Side effects
Isoniazid (INH)	300 mg po	Peripheral neuritis, hepatitis, hypersensitivity
Ethambutol (Myambutol)	25 mg/kg po for 60 days, then 15 mg/kg	Optic neuritis
Rifampin* (Rifadin, Rimactane)	600 mg po	Hepatitis, hypersensitivity reactions
Streptomycin	1 gm IM	Eighth-nerve damage, nephrotoxicity

*Isoniazid and rifampin may be given in combination (Rifamate).

3. Nursing goals

In the case of tuberculosis, it is important to instruct the patient about the disease and how to prevent transmission, ensure adequate room ventilation, collect appropriate sputum specimens, provide oral hygiene and CPT as needed, assess for clinical signs of improvement, provide for adequate nutrition and hydration, assess the emotional response of patient, family, and friends, provide support and encouragement, and instruct the patient about the importance of taking medications for a prolonged period.

QUIZ

1. Match the appropriate assessment findings with each of the pneumonias:

    Pneumococcal _____

    Staphylococcus aureus _____

    Pseudomonas _____

    a. Rusty or greenish sputum, fever with shaking chills, decreased breath sounds

    b. Bradycardia, severe dyspnea, copious yellow or green foul-smelling sputum

    c. Fever, cough that produces purulent material (yellow, brown, or blood-streaked), rales, rhonchi, and decreased breath sounds

2. List five typical assessment findings in a lung abscess patient:

3. An empyema is a collection of infected exudate in the

_____ .

4. List four typical assessment findings in a patient with empyema:

5. What organism causes tuberculosis?

6. The four drugs most commonly used in treating tuberculosis are:

ANSWERS

1. Pneumococcal **a**

 Staphylococcus aureus **c**

 Pseudomonas **b**

2. Low-grade fever, cough with sputum, dyspnea, foul-smelling breath, blood-tinged, purulent, drainage, Anemia and weight loss (if chronic), malaise, dullness to percussion, decreased breath sounds, pleural friction rub, egophony.

3. Pleural space.

4. Elevated temperature, pleural pain, dyspnea, anorexia, leukocytosis, weight loss, absent breath sounds, dullness to percussion, decreased vocal fremitus.

5. *Mycobacterium tuberculosis*.

6. Isoniazid, ethambutol, rifampin, streptomycin.

10

Lung Tumors

OBJECTIVES

After completing this chapter, you will be able to:

1. Identify the most common risk factor in the development of lung cancer

2. List the four major types of lung tumor

3. Explain why the mortality rate is high in lung cancer

4. Identify the most common assessment findings in a lung tumor patient.

A. Introduction

Pulmonary tumors may be benign or malignant; primary or secondary. There are very few benign lung tumors, but those that do exist are usually asymptomatic (except for benign bronchial adenoma, which causes bleeding with hemoptysis). On X-ray, these tumors have clear margins and are well outlined. Whenever possible, they are surgically removed because they can become malignant.

Metastatic, or secondary, tumors often arise from malignant tumors in the breast, stomach, prostate, kidney, thyroid, testis, or bone. Secondary tumors are difficult to differentiate from primary tumors (those that originate in the lungs). It is best to confirm the diagnosis by histologic examination of specimens from bronchial tissue obtained by biopsy or surgical resection.

Most primary tumors develop from the bronchial epithelium and are malignant (they are called bronchogenic carcinoma). These tumors are usually on the right side and located centrally rather than on the periphery of the lung. Because of their proximity to the mediastinum, they are often inoperable. If untreated, however, bronchogenic carcinoma is fatal within 9 months.

B. Classification

The most common type of primary pulmonary carcinoma is squamous cell (epidermoid) carcinoma. It usually develops in the main bronchi or larger bronchial branches. Primary lung tumors may metastasize to the brain, adrenal glands, liver, bones, and opposite lung. The four main types of invasive lung cancer are epidermoid carcinoma, small-cell anaplastic carcinoma, adenocarcinoma, and large-cell carcinoma.

C. Incidence and etiology

Lung cancer is the number one cause of cancer deaths among men in the United States and it has steadily been increasing among women as well. The mortality rate is high because it is difficult to diagnose at an early stage. However, most types of lung cancer can be cured if detected early enough. Lung cancer is largely preventable because it is typically caused by cigarette smoking. The risk of getting lung cancer increases in proportion to the number of cigarettes smoked, how long the individual has smoked, how deeply the smoker inhales, and the age at which he began. Other risk factors for lung cancer include uranium mining, exposure to asbestos, working with chromate or arsenic, exposure to bischloromethyl ether, previous upper respiratory tract cancer, and air pollution.

D. Assessment

In the early stages, lung cancer is usually detectable only by chest X-ray. By the time symptoms appear, the cancer may be so advanced that it is beyond the possibility of cure. The most common symptom of bronchogenic carcinoma is the appearance of a cough (in 90 percent of those affected) or a change in the nature of the cough (becomes persistent).

Other symptoms include hemoptysis, chest pain (late), symptoms of pulmonary infection, wheezing (when a bronchus becomes partially obstructed by the tumor), weight loss, fatigue, and anorexia.

E. Treatment

Treatment will vary according to the cell type and stage of the disease. The four approaches are surgery, radiation, chemotherapy, and immunotherapy.

F. Nursing goals

It is important to assist the patient through his treatment, educate the patient about the side effects of radiation therapy and chemotherapy, provide for comfort and the relief of pain, maintain adequate ventilation and airway patency, provide adequate nutrition and hydration, and support the patient and his family emotionally in confronting a possible terminal illness.

QUIZ

1. The most common risk factor in the development of lung cancer is _____ .

2. List the four major types of lung tumor:

3. Lung cancer has a high mortality rate because the diagnosis is usually made _____ in the illness.

4. The most common assessment finding in broncho-genic carcinoma is _____ .

ANSWERS
1. Smoking.
2. Epidermoid carcinoma, small-cell anaplastic carcinoma, adeno-carcinoma, large-cell carcinoma.
3. Late.
4. Cough.

11

Chest Trauma

OBJECTIVES

After completing this chapter, you will be able to:

1. Make an immediate assessment of the patient with chest trauma

2. Specify the four classifications of injury to the chest

3. Describe three types of chest trauma and list at least two assessment findings for each.

A. Introduction

Thoracic injuries are usually obvious and therefore can be treated early with generally excellent results. The major causes of thoracic injury are auto accidents, industrial accidents, knives, and low-velocity bullets.

B. Immediate assessment

The first priority in chest trauma is to ensure adequate ventilation. This would include maintaining a patent airway and perhaps assisting ventilation. Begin with the ABCs of cardiopulmonary resuscitation (CPR) — airway, breathing, circulation. Next, determine if there is an airway obstruction, massive pneumo- or hemothorax, or open chest wound. Then, if it is feasible, take a brief history of the incident and make a quick assessment of the type of injury sustained.

C. Classification

1. Blunt trauma (nonpenetrating)

This type of injury is caused by forceful contact with a blunt object (such as a steering wheel) and is often associated with serious intracranial or abdominal injury. The chest wall is affected, but not the pleural cavity or lung tissue. Blunt trauma may occur in automobile accidents, falls, assaults, or explosions.

2. Penetrating

These wounds, involving the chest wall and pleural cavity, are caused by high-velocity missiles or sharp objects.

3. Perforating

These wounds are through and through (there is an entrance and an exit). In a gunshot wound, the exit wound is usually larger and more ragged because the bullet has tumbled or changed during passage through the body tissues.

4. Open/closed

In an open wound there is a constant exchange of air between the atmosphere and the pleural cavity. In a closed wound, there is no communication between the pleural cavity and the atmosphere.

D. Rib fracture

This is the most common type of chest trauma and usually involves the third to 10th ribs because they are less protected by other structures.

1. Assessment

The patient with rib fracture will have distinct symptoms, such as pain with movement of the rib cage, splinting with movement of the rib cage, dyspnea, tenderness and swelling, and ecchymosis. If there is a suspected first-rib fracture, look for neck injuries, brachial plexus injuries, pneumothorax, or aortic tear.

2. Treatment

The following measures are recommended: intercostal nerve block, analgesics (especially before therapy), no taping of the chest, and bronchial hygiene.

E. Flail chest

This injury occurs when there are multiple fractures of ribs on the same side, a fracture of the sternum, or fracture of a rib in at least two places. Because a section of the thorax is not supported by a competent bony structure, there is paradoxical movement of the chest wall in that area. Such instability can cause hypoventilation, hypoxia, and hypercapnia. It may be associated with a lung contusion.

1. Assessment

The symptoms that are typical of this injury include rapid, shallow respirations, cyanosis, tachycardia, paradoxical chest movement, shock, severe chest wall pain, and bony crepitus at flail.

2. Treatment

As soon as flail chest is recognized, pressure is applied over the flail segment, using sandbags, adhesive, or hands. Later, internal fixation is accomplished by intubation and mechanical ventilation for 7 to 10 days or longer.

F. Pneumothorax

After a penetrating wound to the chest wall, the pleural cavity loses its negative pressure and the lung collapses.

1. Assessment

Among patients with pneumothorax, you will probably note increased chest pain, dyspnea, decreased or absent breath sounds on affected side, hyperresonance on percussion, and shock.

2. Treatment

Apply an occlusive pressure dressing (Vaseline-impregnated gauze) if there is an open wound. Chest tubes and underwater-seal drainage are used to drain air in the pleural cavity.

G. Tension pneumothorax

This type of lung collapse is created by a pleural tear with ball-valve action. Air can be sucked in on inspiration, but the tear closes on expiration, trapping the air inside the lung cavity. The space fills with air, which then begins to press on the opposite side, the mediastinum, and the heart. This life-threatening condition requires immediate action.

1. Assessment

You may be able to observe the following: respiratory distress, tracheal shift away from the affected side, mediastinal shift away from the affected side, hyperresonance on percussion of the affected side, decreased or absent breath sounds on the affected side, and shift of the point of maximal impulse (PMI) away from the affected side.

2. Treatment

As an emergency measure, to allow air to escape from the pleural cavity, a large-bore needle may be inserted in the second or third intercostal space at the midclavicular line. Later, chest tubes with underwater-seal drainage are inserted.

H. Hemothorax

This is a pneumothorax with a laceration of the lung tissue or intercostal artery. Gravity causes blood to accumulate at the bottom of the lungs.

1. Assessment

The patient with hemothorax will probably exhibit respiratory distress, dullness to percussion where fluid collects, absent or distant breath sounds, fever, and shock (if hemorrhage is extensive).

2. Treatment

The following measures may be taken: thoracocentesis or chest tube drainage, replacement of the lost blood, autotransfusion (if there is massive hemorrhaging), direct repair of the bleeding vessel, and antibiotics if infection develops.

I. Contusion of the lung

Bruising or hemorrhage into the lung parenchyma and alveoli results in severe V/Q abnormalities with accompanying pneumonia. ARDS is a common sequela to this type of severe lung injury.

1. Assessment

It is important to look for the following: increased secretions, hemoptysis (which is usually present), increased fluid in interstitium, intrapulmonary shunting, decreased compliance, and increased work of breathing.

2. Treatment

Treating lung contusions usually consists of mechanical ventilation, CPT, including postural drainage, close monitoring and relief of pain.

J. Cardiac tamponade

Defined as compression of the heart by blood or fluid in the pericardial sac, cardiac tamponade is often caused by a penetrating wound. It may develop within hours or minutes.

1. Assessment

The following symptoms may be observed in the cardiac tamponade patient: distended neck veins, elevated central venous pressure (CVP), muffled or distant heart sounds, shock, narrow pulse pressure, and pulsus paradoxus.

2. Treatment

Therapeutic approaches include pericardial aspiration, thoracotomy, pericardiotomy, and direct repair of the wound.

K. Diaphragmatic injuries

Such injuries involve either the rupture or herniation of the diaphragm. They occur more frequently on the left than on the right side because the right side is protected by the liver.

1. Assessment

You may note any of these typical symptoms: respiratory distress, referred shoulder pain on the same side as the tear, inability to insert a nasogastric tube, decreased P_aO_2 and increased P_aCO_2, signs of cardiorespiratory collapse, and elevated hemidiaphragm on X-ray.

2. Treatment

There are two therapeutic approaches: surgical repair of the tear and provision of ventilatory support.

L. Fracture of trachea or bronchus

Although rare, this type of injury is associated with severe chest trauma and fracture of the upper ribs. It results in escape of air into the chest cavity, which can cause pneumothorax as well as mediastinal and subcutaneous emphysema. It is diagnosed by bronchoscopy.

1. Assessment

Symptoms typically occurring in a patient with this injury are cough, bloody sputum, respiratory distress, and subcutaneous emphysema.

2. Treatment

The following modes of therapy are recommended: intubation, mechanical ventilation, operative repair.

QUIZ

1. The first priority in caring for a patient with chest trauma is to maintain adequate _____.

2. The four classifications of chest trauma are:

3. Match each assessment finding with the appropriate chest trauma:

Paradoxical chest motion _____

Tenderness, swelling _____

Tracheal shift away from affected side _____

Pain with breathing _____

Hyperresonance on percussion _____

Bony crepitus _____

Shoulder pain on affected side _____

Inability to insert nasogastric tube _____

a. Rib fracture

b. Tension pneumothorax

c. Flail chest

d. Diaphragmatic injuries

1. Ventilation.

2. Blunt, penetrating, perforating, open/closed.

3. Paradoxical chest motion **c**.
   Tenderness, swelling **a**.
   Tracheal shift away from affected side **b**.
   Pain with breathing **a**.
   Hyperresonance on percussion **b**.
   Bony crepitus **c**.
   Shoulder pain on affected side **d**.
   Inability to insert NG tube **d**.

12

Acute Respiratory Failure and Adult Respiratory Distress Syndrome

OBJECTIVES

After completing this chapter, you will be able to:

1. *Differentiate between acute respiratory failure (ARF) and adult respiratory distress syndrome (ARDS)*

2. *Recognize the patient who is at high risk of developing ARF and ARDS*

3. *Identify the signs and symptoms of ARF and ARDS, and list three therapeutic goals for each*

4. *Explain positive end-expiratory pressure (PEEP) and its effect on the respiratory system.*

A. Introduction

ARF and ARDS are two umbrella terms for common physiologic changes occurring in the lung regardless of etiology. This author views ARF as a general condition, and ARDS as a subtype with its own specific pathophysiologic changes. Although closely related, the two conditions will be discussed separately here.

B. ARF

1. Definition

Also known as ventilatory failure, this condition exists when the P_aO_2 is 50 mm Hg or less and/or the P_aCO_2 is 50 mm Hg or more. Regardless of the underlying cause (e.g., pneumonia), the patient will manifest the signs and symptoms of hypoxemia and/or hypercapnia. The goals of management are to correct these two problems as well as to treat the underlying cause.

2. Etiology and precipitating causes

Almost any lung condition, if severe enough, will produce ARF. Probably the most common cause is alveolar hypoven-

TABLE 12-1

COMMON CAUSES OF ARF

Causes	Clinical features
Drug overdose	Coma
Infection	↑ Secretions, ↓ VC
Neuromuscular diseases	
Myasthenia gravis	↓ VC
Guillain-Barré syndrome	↓ VC
Poliomyelitis	Irregular respirations
Muscular dystrophy	Myotonia
Head injury	Apnea or depressed respirations
Chest trauma	Flail chest, respiratory distress
COPD	↓ FEV_1, possibly ↑ secretions
Surgery	↓ VC
Burns	↓ VC, laryngotracheal edema
Obesity	↓ VC

tilation due to COPD. Table 12-1 presents typical causes of ARF and their major clinical features.

3. Pathophysiology

The alveolar hypoventilation that results in ARF is due to abnormal distribution of inspired gases, which may be caused by dead space ventilation, decreased respiratory drive, mucus plugging, lung tissue injury, alveolar destruction, interstitial fluid, or inadequate movement of the chest wall. Blood flow is adequate and the diffusion of gases across the alveolar-capillary membrane is normal. However, intrapulmonary shunting is common because the blood flow exceeds ventilation, and the blood returning to the heart is unoxygenated; thus, there is venous admixture and hypoxemia (Figure 12-1). The outcome is respiratory acidosis.

4. Clinical picture and nursing assessment

Because ARF results from impaired alveolar gas exchange, the main clinical finding is abnormal arterial blood gas values, increased P_aCO_2 and decreased P_aO_2. Hypercapnia develops only when there is hypoventilation and/or $\dot{V}/\dot{Q}$ mismatching. Hypoxemia without hypercapnia develops when the capillary bed is reduced or the alveolar-capillary membrane is thickened. Table 12-2 presents the signs and symptoms of hypoxia and hypercapnia.

Figure 12-1 *Physiologic stages of acute respiratory failure. Adapted, with permission, from Cherniack RM et al: Respiration in Health and Disease, ed 2. Philadelphia, WB Saunders, 1972, p 435.*

↑ Work of breathing

↑ O_2 consumption   ↓ V_T P_aCO_2 Hypoxemia   Hypoxia

Hypercapnia

Alveolar hypoventilation	Venous admixture	Dead space ventilation
	Uneven ventilation and perfusion	
Respiratory depression	Pulmonary disease	Chest wall disease

TABLE 12-2

CLINICAL SIGNS AND SYMPTOMS OF ARF

Hypoxia	*Hypercapnia*
Confusion	Drowsiness/somnolence
Restlessness/anxiety	Headache
Loss of judgment	Personality changes
Dizziness	Coma
Unconsciousness	Pink, warm skin
Sympathetic responses	Papilledema
Tachycardia	Diaphoresis
Cold, pale skin	Asterixis (flopping tremor)
Nonsympathetic responses	Hypertension (systemic and pulmonary)
Bradycardia	Tachycardia
Hypotension	Dyspnea and tachypnea
Tachyarrhythmias	Wheezes
Central cyanosis	
Dyspnea	

Because these clinical findings will vary from patient to patient, depending on the underlying disorder and its severity, you need to be alert to the variations. Early manifestations of ARF include the cerebral signs of anxiety, restlessness, dyspnea, and headache. You may also note a gradual increase in blood pressure and pulse rates; shallow, rapid respirations; inability to speak three or four words without gasping; use of the accessory muscles of respiration; asymmetrical movement of the chest with deep breaths; diaphoresis; and rales or wheezes. Later cerebral manifestations are somnolence, mental confusion, papilledema, and coma.

5. Treatment

Emphasis should be placed on managing the patient aggressively so he will not need mechanical ventilatory support. Although the patient may be cared for on a medical-surgical floor, often it is better for him to be in an intensive care unit, which can provide constant observation and assessment, has complex monitoring and mechanical equipment, and can deal with respiratory emergencies.

Besides treating the underlying disorder, the main goals of therapy are as follows:

a. Maintain adequate oxygenation

- Give oxygen, with the specific amount depending on level of hypoxemia (low-flow O_2 if patient is chronically hypercapnic)
- Monitor effectiveness of therapy (look for signs of hypoxia)
- Support the circulatory system (if blood is not being pumped adequately) with digoxin, diuretics, vasopressors, or fluids
- Perform phlebotomy if the hematocrit is above 60 percent and blood is "sluggish"
- Limit activity (activity increases O_2 demand on the lungs).

b. Maintain effective tracheobronchial hygiene

- Combat bronchospasm with bronchodilators and steroids intravenously and by nebulization
- Provide for inhalation of moisture
- Clear the airway by tracheal suction or by encouraging the patient to cough
- Use postural drainage, percussion, and vibration to help mobilize secretions.

c. Control alveolar ventilation. The measures just outlined may correct hypoventilation. In addition:

- Periodic IPPB treatments may improve ventilation
- Endotracheal intubation and mechanical ventilation may be needed if hypoventilation is not corrected by other means.

d. Combat bronchopulmonary infections

- Obtain culture samples periodically for identification of specific organism(s)
- Administer antibiotic therapy as ordered.

C. ARDS

This syndrome is an acute, life-threatening lung condition that has any number of causes. By definition it is a form of ARF because it is characterized by hypoxemia (and, later in its course, by hypercapnia). Whatever the cause, the patho-physiologic changes are the same and treatment needs to be directed toward those changes.

Since ARDS patients are probably the sickest respiratory patients, they are usually managed in critical care units. Wherever you work, however, it is important to have the assessment skills and be able to recognize the early signs of ARDS because early detection dramatically increases the patient's chances to survive.

1. Definition

ARDS, also known as shock lung, is an umbrella term that covers many clinical, pathologic, and physiologic abnormalities. It usually results from shock or a shock-like state, and what we see are the effects of hypoperfusion on the lungs. However, since the symptoms may not appear until hours or days after the precipitating incident, you should be able to recognize those patients who are at high risk of developing ARDS and be alert to the evolving clinical signs. Table 12-3 lists the disorders associated with ARDS.

2. Pathophysiology

The physiologic chain of events begins with shock and leads to pulmonary hypoperfusion; this, in turn, leads to edema, atelectasis, and ultimately hypoxemia (see Figure 12-2).

When shock reduces the normal blood flow to the lungs, both the alveolar and the capillary endothelium are injured. As a consequence, platelets aggregate in the pulmonary capillaries, leading to the formation of multiple microthrombi and the release of vasoactive substances that produce further injury. The capillary membrane becomes abnormally permeable, promoting leakage of plasma and proteins from the capillaries into the interstitial spaces, alveoli, and bronchioles (this fluid accumulation is known as noncardiogenic pulmonary edema). Leaking of plasma proteins may also cause the formation of hyaline membranes.

Because of injury to the alveolar wall from hypoperfusion and edema, type II pneumocytes are damaged and the production of surfactant is impaired. The decrease in surfac-

TABLE 12-3

PRECIPITATING CAUSES OF ARDS

Shock (from any cause)
Infections
    Viral pneumonia
    Gram-negative sepsis
    Bacterial pneumonia
    Fungal pneumonia
Trauma
    Multisystem
    Fat embolus
    Lung contusion (flail chest)
    Nonthoracic trauma (including head injury)
Drug overdose
Toxic inhalations
    O_2 toxicity
    Smoke inhalation
    Corrosive chemicals (NO_2, Cl_2, NH_3, phosgene)
Hematologic disorders
    Disseminated intravascular coagulation (DIC)
    Massive blood transfusions
    Postperfusion (cardiopulmonary bypass)
Liquid aspiration
    Gastric juice
    Near drowning
    Hydrocarbon fluids (kerosene, gasoline)
Metabolic disorders
    Pancreatitis
    Uremia
Fluid overload
Sepsis

tant causes atelectasis of alveoli that are not filled with fluid. The end result is impaired gas exchange, intrapulmonary shunting, and decreased compliance.

Initially the patient will hyperventilate in an attempt to take in more oxygen. But this maneuver actually blows off carbon dioxide, producing hypocapnia. Hyperventilation usually does not improve the oxygen level in these patients, and hypoxemia continues.

3. Clinical picture and nursing assessment

The clinical manifestation has three stages. During the earliest stage (after the initial shocklike injury), there may be no

Figure 12-2 *Physiologic stages of ARDS. Adapted, with permission, from Hopewell PC: Adult respiratory distress syndrome. Basics of RD, ATS News, Summer 1979, p 16.*

Trauma, infection, other causes		Pulmonary hypoperfusion, hypoxemia
Alveolar-capillary membrane injury		
Increased alveolar and capillary wall permeability	Microvascular thrombi and platelet aggregation	Damage to type II pneumocyte
Stagnation of blood, release of injury agents	Leakage of fluid and proteins into tissues	Decreased surfactant
Interstitial and alveolar edema (noncardiogenic pulmonary edema)	Alveolar and/or airway filling or closure	
Reduced FRC, intrapulmonary shunting, reduced compliance		
Atelectasis Hypoxemia		
Hyperventilation (hypocapnia)		Hypoventilation (hypercapnia)

evidence of respiratory dysfunction unless the injury is severe, there is major lung involvement, or there is pre-existing lung dysfunction. Even without clear-cut findings, you should recognize those who are at high risk and look for subtle changes in their orientation, mood, and personality as well as note any increase in temperature, pulse, and respirations.

During the second stage — the progression of hypocapnia and hypoxemia, which may occur 24 to 48 hours after the initial injury — you will observe dyspnea with suprasternal and intercostal retractions, flaring of the nares, and grunting respirations. The patient will be cyanotic, have rales and rhonchi on auscultation, and exhibit tachycardia, diaphoresis, and confusion. A chest X-ray will show cloudy infiltrates in all lung fields, suggestive of pulmonary edema. At this point, oxygen therapy will be either ordered or increased, but the hypoxemia will continue because of the worsening gas exchange. Blood gas tests will reveal hypoxemia, respiratory alkalosis, and metabolic acidosis (from hypoxia). Thus, a hallmark of ARDS is a decreasing P_aO_2 despite attempts to increase the fraction of inspired oxygen (F_iO_2).

Even when high concentrations of oxygen are used, the patient's condition will continue to deteriorate. Eventually, if ARDS is identified too late and not corrected, the last stage will be reached, in which the patient won't be able to compensate by hyperventilation. At that point, CO_2 retention and respiratory acidosis will ensue.

4. Treatment

The main focus should be on prevention. The underlying cause of the hypoperfusion to the lung should be treated. Treating the hypotension as well would require volume replacement and vasoactive drugs. Patients sustaining a hypoperfusion incident should be treated in intensive care. The goals of therapy are to: increase oxygen to the tissues, increase P_aO_2 (initially), and decrease the patient's oxygen consumption.

a. Fluid management. Because of increased capillary permeability, giving excessive fluids, especially during resuscitation, can aggravate or produce pulmonary edema. But, too little fluid replacement will result in inadequate pulmonary and systemic perfusion. Therefore, volume replacement must be done carefully and monitored closely.

Monitoring is best achieved with the tip of a flow-directed (Swan-Ganz) catheter in a branch of the pulmonary artery. This measures pulmonary artery wedge pressure (PAWP), which reflects left ventricular function. With the catheter in place, fluids can be administered to maintain perfusion to the vital organs without taxing the heart unduly. If the PAWP increases before there is adequate perfusion, vasopressors may be required.

The catheter also permits measurement of mixed venous blood in order to assess systemic tissue oxygenation, and measurement of cardiac output directly by the thermal dilution method.

In giving fluids to those with ARDS, it is probably best to give crystalloids initially when the capillaries are most permeable and protein and plasma are leaking. Later on, colloids (protein substances) should be used, especially if the serum protein concentration is low.

b. Ventilatory support. It is difficult to decide exactly when to provide ventilatory support to patients at risk for ARDS. To forestall a vicious cycle of edema and lung volume loss leading to more edema, more volume loss, and severe hypoxia, it is preferable to intubate and mechanically ventilate these patients earlier rather than later (see Chapter 15). With mechanical ventilation, large tidal volumes of 10 to 15 ml/kg body weight should be used because they are more effective in preventing or reversing atelectasis. Occasionally, added dead space will be needed to correct for the hyperventilation that usually coincides with large tidal volumes.

c. PEEP. In ARDS many factors contribute to a decrease in lung volume. PEEP overcomes these factors by producing a constant positive distending pressure across the walls of the airways and alveoli. PEEP is achieved by adjusting a valve on a volume ventilator so that positive pressure is applied at the end of expiration and the pressure does not return to zero with each breath. This pressure opens closed alveoli and prevents others from becoming atelectatic. Consequently, functional residual capacity (FRC) is increased and oxygenation is improved (by increasing the P_aO_2). PEEP may also help push some of the fluid out of the alveoli, thereby improving gas exchange.

With the improvement in P_aO_2, less oxygen usually needs to be delivered, making oxygen toxicity less likely. Since PEEP increases FRC, it will improve lung compliance. PEEP may also conserve surfactant, further improving lung compliance.

The major complications occurring with PEEP are decreased cardiac output (elevated airway pressure in the chest is transmitted to the great vessels, resulting in decreased venous return to the heart) and pneumothorax (from overdistention and rupture of less diseased alveoli).

d. Corticosteroids. Although their use is controversial, steroids may decrease edema by stabilizing the lysosomal membranes (which could otherwise produce lung injury) and by reducing the fibrosis that could occur after the acute phase of the illness.

D. Nursing diagnoses and management

Patients with both ARF and ARDS require frequent monitoring and assessment of their status. As the patient's condition worsens, the complexity and amount of nursing care required increase. You may be called upon simply to administer oxygen therapy and bronchodilators, or you may need to perform mechanical ventilation with PEEP and monitor pulmonary artery pressures.

General nursing guidelines for these patients include: maintenance of adequate airway patency; ensuring adequate oxygenation and ventilation, keeping P_aO_2 and P_aCO_2 levels within normal limits; ensuring adequate oxygenation and perfusion of organs and tissues; prevention of infection and other complications; alleviation of the patient's and family's anxiety by explaining the disease process, diagnostic procedures, and treatment plans; maintenance of hemodynamic stability; and treating the underlying disease condition.

QUIZ

1. In ARF, the P_aO_2 is _____ and the P_aCO_2 is _____ .

2. ARDS usually develops because of a period of _____ _____ in the lung.

3. List three precipitating causes for ARF and three for ARDS:

4. Indicate if the following assessment findings are present in ARF, ARDS, or both:

Hypoxemia _____

Rib retractions _____

Cloudy infiltrates on chest X-ray _____

Shallow, rapid respirations _____

Papilledema _____

Wheezes _____

Rales _____

Confusion _____

5. List three treatments for ARF and ARDS:

6. PEEP is effective in treating ARDS because it provides a constant _____ , thereby improving _____ .

ANSWERS

1. ≤ 50 mm Hg; ≥ 50 mm Hg.

2. Hypoperfusion.

3. ARF: drug overdose, infections, COPD, neuromuscular diseases, head injury, chest trauma, surgery, burns, obesity.

ARDS: shock, infections, trauma, drug overdose, hematologic disorders, aspiration, metabolic disorders, fluid overload, sepsis.

4. Hypoxemia both.   Papilledema ARF.

Rib retractions ARDS.   Wheezes ARF.

Cloudy infiltrates on chest X-ray ARDS.   Rales both.

Shallow, rapid respirations both.   Confusion both.

5. ARF: adequate oxygenation, tracheobronchial hygiene, ventilatory support, treat infections.

ARDS: fluid management, ventilatory support, use of PEEP, steroids.

6. Positive distending pressure; oxygenation.

13

Airway Management

OBJECTIVES

After completing this chapter, you will be able to:

1. *List two indications for the use of an oral airway, nasal airway, endotracheal tube, and tracheostomy tube*

2. *Describe the characteristics of a tracheostomy tube*

3. *List five potential complications of prolonged tracheostomy tube placement*

4. *State the optimal cuff pressure range and demonstrate how to measure cuff pressure.*

A. Pharyngeal airways

1. Oropharyngeal airway

This airway, which conforms to the shape of the palate and extends into the pharynx, is used to keep the tongue down, to prevent the patient from biting down (on an endotracheal tube or his tongue), and to facilitate the removal of secretions. To insert the oral airway, open the patient's mouth with your index finger and thumb crossed and rotate the airway as you insert it over the tongue (Figure 13-1). When the airway is in place, secure it with tape.

Oral airways come in many sizes. They permit air to pass around and through them. Good mouth care is essential. Remember, though, that this type of airway does not guarantee airflow. If the patient is apneic, hyperextend his neck using the head tilt/chin lift method and deliver mouth-to-mouth breathing until help arrives.

2. Nasopharyngeal airway

This is a soft, latex, catheter-like tube that is inserted through the nose (Figure 13-2). It is especially helpful when frequent

Figure 13-1 *Oropharyngeal airway*

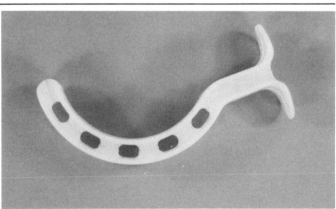

Figure 13-2 *Nasopharyngeal airway*

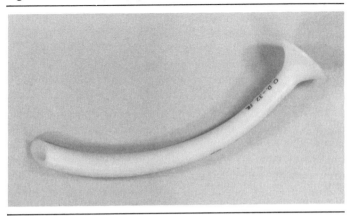

"blind" suctioning is required. It will serve as a guide to positioning a suction catheter just above the epiglottis and will minimize any irritation to the mucosa in the nose from frequent suctioning.

Available in various sizes, this tube extends from the nostril to just below the base of the tongue. It's inserted by lubricating the tip with a water-soluble lubricant and gently pushing the tube through the entire length of the nostril. This airway does not prevent a patient with an oral endotracheal tube from biting down and occluding the tube.

The airway should be changed from nostril to nostril every 8 hours, and the area cleaned each time.

B. Endotracheal tubes

1. Indications

These tubes are used in almost any emergency calling for intubation, and also in nonemergent situations when a tube will be required only briefly. Endotracheal intubation avoids the complications of surgical tracheostomy. If functioning properly, endotracheal tubes may safely remain in place for up to 3 weeks.

2. Characteristics

Endotracheal tubes are made of polyvinyl chloride, which is soft and pliable, and are disposable. They have a large, low-pressure cuff that is inflated to maintain a seal for ventilation and to prevent aspiration. They all have a 15-mm universal adapter that fits on the end of the tube and can readily be attached to a ventilator, resuscitation bag, aerosol tubing, etc.

Oral endotracheal tubes have several advantages over nasal endotracheal tubes: they are larger and thus are preferable for ventilation and removal of secretions; they can be shifted from side to side in the mouth, thereby avoiding excessive irritation and pressure; and they are easier to insert.

On the other hand, nasal endotracheal tubes are generally more comfortable for patients, as it's possible to mouth words and, sometimes, to eat with these tubes in place. Patients cannot bite down on these tubes too easily and so are less likely to obstruct them. However, these tubes must be relatively small in diameter so that they can be inserted through the nose (which increases the chance of obstruction due to secretions), and they are not easily changed from one nostril to another. If a patient needs an endotracheal tube for 2 or 3 weeks, the oral tube is preferable.

3. Intubation

Although this procedure is usually not performed by nurses in hospitals, you will need to make sure that the necessary equipment is available and functioning. Every unit should have an intubation tray holding various-sized tubes as well as laryngoscope blades, laryngoscope handle with extra bulbs and batteries, lubricant, guide wire, lidocaine (Xylocaine) spray, tape, and syringes. Suction catheters and a suction unit should also be available, for you will need to suction the patient before and after intubation or as indicated by the physician.

Before the tube is inserted, you should also make sure that the cuff inflates symmetrically and has no leak. Once the tube is in place, you should remind the physician to order a postintubation chest X-ray to verify its placement and then tape the tube securely in place.

4. Complications

Major complications include vocal cord damage on intubation or extubation, absence of cough or gag reflex initially, large airway resistance, inadvertent extubation, and swallowing dysfunction.

5. Extubation

The criteria for this procedure include response of the patient to oral commands, a VC of more than 10 ml/kg of body weight, ability to generate a maximum inspiratory force of more than -20 cm H_2O, and satisfactory ABGs as determined by the physician.

After the criteria have been met and an order written, the patient should be extubated (see Table 13-1) and placed on oxygen and humidification (usually an aerosol mask).

C. Tracheostomy tubes

1. Indications

A tracheostomy should never be performed on an emergency basis except in the case of severe facial injuries, facial burns, or complete upper airway obstruction (such as epiglottitis). A tracheostomy is appropriate for patients with upper airway obstruction, those having extensive face and neck surgery, those who need ventilatory assistance for a

TABLE 13-1

STEPS IN EXTUBATION PROCEDURE

Suction airway thoroughly
Deflate endotracheal tube cuff
Reinsert suction catheter without applying suction
Ask patient to exhale or cough gently
As he exhales or coughs, pull out the tube, suctioning as you go to remove secretions
Assist patient in coughing up excess secretions
Immediately place patient on humidification and oxygenation source (as ordered)
Look for stridor and increasing respiratory distress, which indicate patient's need to be reintubated

prolonged period, those who need long-term airway management (stroke and comatose patients), and those who might aspirate oral/gastric secretions.

2. Characteristics

These tubes are similar to endotracheal tubes except for their size and shape. They vary in size, some have inner cannulas, and there are different methods for maintaining cuff pressure. It is important for you to know if your patient has an inner-cannula tube because the inner cannula requires additional care.

Although the cuffs of all disposable tracheostomy tubes are low pressure, some require a constant volume of air and equalize the pressure with the external balloon, some have a pressure relief valve, and one has a foam cuff where only ambient air fills the balloon. Most have a conventional cuff with a one-way valve to seal in the air used to inflate the cuff. There are also tubes without cuffs, with fenestrations, and with other features that are helpful in weaning the patient from a tracheostomy tube. Figure 13-3 illustrates the types of tubes available and Table 13-2 details when they should be utilized.

3. Tracheostomy procedure

Since this is a surgical procedure, it is usually performed in the operating room. However, in some critical care units as well as emergency departments, it may be performed at the bedside. It is important to try to maintain a sterile environment as much as possible throughout the procedure.

4. Complications

Complications may occur during any of the following three periods: *Immediately after the procedure*, there may be bleeding, pneumothorax, air embolism, aspiration, subcutaneous or mediastinal emphysema, recurrent laryngeal nerve damage, or posterior tracheal wall penetration. *Over weeks or years*, the patient may experience airway obstruction secondary to secretions or cuff over the tip of the tube, infection, rupture of the brachiocephalic trunk (innominate artery), dysphagia, tracheoesophageal fistula, tracheal dilation, or

Figure 13-3 *Varieties of tracheostomy tubes. Upper row, from left to right: Shiley tube with disposable inner cannula; Shiley tube with single cannula; Portex tube with single cannula. Lower row, from left to right: cuffless tube; fenestrated tube with cuff; fenestrated tube without cuff*

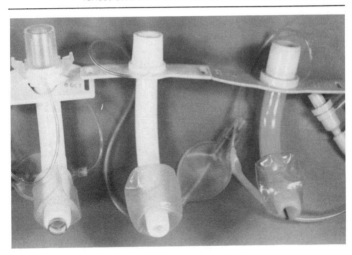

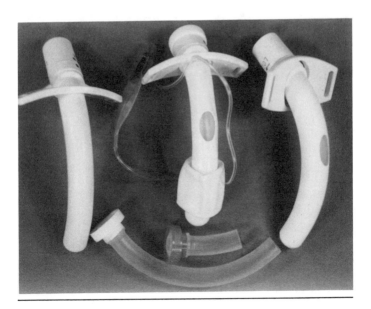

TABLE 13-2

TYPES AND USES OF TRACHEOSTOMY TUBES

Type	Indications
Cuffed with inner cannula	Decreased level of consciousness, tube feedings, fresh tracheostomy, mechanical ventilation
Cuffed without inner cannula	Decreased level of consciousness, tube feedings, fresh tracheostomy, mechanical ventilation
Cuffless	Conscious, spontaneous breathing; some airflow to upper airway
Fenestrated with cuff	Weaning from trach, greater airflow across upper airway, in an emergency can be converted and patient placed back on ventilator
Fenestrated without cuff	Weaning, greater airflow across airway
Trach button	Maintains stoma, does not enter trachea, permanent tracheostomy, can be plugged when not needed

tracheal ischemia and necrosis. *After the tube is removed,* the patient may suffer acute airway obstruction, tracheal stenosis, or vocal cord paralysis (secondary to laryngeal nerve damage).

D. Endotracheal versus tracheostomy tubes

Table 13-3 highlights the characteristics of these two types of airways.

E. Cuff management

1. Indications for cuff inflation

As a general rule the cuff on a tracheostomy tube should be deflated. It should be inflated only for the following reasons: when continuous ventilation is needed, during and 1 hour after eating (or tube feeding), during IPPB treatments, when the patient cannot handle oral secretions, or when there is danger of aspiration (e.g., the unconscious patient who has little or no cough reflex).

Once a cuff has been inflated, however, it remains that way. It should generally be deflated once each hospital shift in order to remove secretions that have collected above the cuff and to measure the cuff pressure. (Deflating cuffs for 5 minutes every hour has been found to be ineffective.)

2. Characteristics of low-pressure cuffs

The cuffs on endotracheal and tracheostomy tubes today have certain features that have significantly reduced the incidence of long-term complications: They can hold large volumes; they have low intracuff pressures at occluding volumes; they are floppy and easily distensible; and they adapt to the tracheal contour, continuing to maintain a seal while exerting minimal pressure on the mucosa.

3. Inflating and measuring cuff pressures

The key to inflating a cuff is to keep the pressure exerted on the tracheal wall below capillary pressure (which is around 27 cm H_2O or 17 mm Hg). The cuff should be inflated until a

TABLE 13-3

COMPARING ENDOTRACHEAL AND TRACHEOSTOMY TUBES

Item	Endotracheal tubes	Tracheostomy tubes
Time required for placement	1-2 min	15 min
Personnel required for placement	Trained RN or paramedic	Surgeon
Duration of use	1-21 days	Indefinite
Removal of secretions	Harder to do (longer, narrower tubes)	Readily achieved
Patient tolerance	Cannot talk, cannot swallow, uncomfortable	Requires psychological adjustment
Nursing care	More difficult	Accessible
Positioning problem	May enter one bronchus only	Usually minor
Replacement	Requires trained personnel	Readily done
Fixation	Requires careful anchoring	Readily done

Figure 13-4 *Cuff pressure gauge*

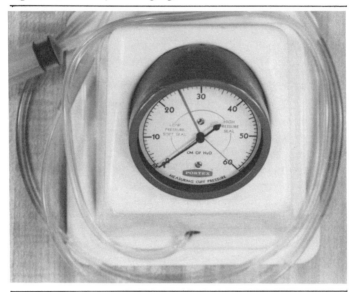

seal is established. The volume of air needed to inflate the cuff should be documented, but it is not as important as the cuff pressure and will vary considerably from patient to patient. The optimal cuff pressure is 15 to 25 cm H_2O (12 to 20 mm Hg). The gauge for measuring cuff pressure is attached to the system (see Figure 13-4), and the pressure needed to seal the airway should be monitored. Table 13-4 explains the technique.

F. Suctioning

This is a sterile procedure that requires meticulous care in order to minimize complications and maximize effectiveness. You will have to judge when to suction a patient; it will depend on the amount of secretions and the patient's condition. Table 13-5 explains the procedure for blind intratracheal suctioning, and Table 13-6 describes how to suction through an endotracheal or tracheostomy tube.

TABLE 13-4

MINIMAL CUFF INFLATION AND
CUFF PRESSURE MEASUREMENT TECHNIQUE

Deflate cuff completely

Connect pressure gauge and 10-ml syringe via three-way stopcock

Slowly inject 1 ml of air at a time into the cuff during inspiration
(positive pressure phase), using a manual resuscitator bag or a
mechanical ventilator

Listen for air (a gurgling sound) with the stethoscope placed on one
side of the neck. If gurgling is present, more air is needed to
create a seal

A seal is created when the gurgling disappears, no air leaks from the
nose and mouth, or the conscious patient cannot make a sound

Note and record the volume and pressure required to seal the cuff

---

G. Tracheostomy care

Care of a patient with a single-cannula tube or a double-cannula tube with a disposable inner cannula involves cleaning the tracheostomy site with hydrogen peroxide and rinsing it with sterile water, then applying a fresh dressing and tapes. If the inner cannula is nondisposable, you'll have to clean it as well.

With a fresh tracheostomy, care generally is required every 2 to 4 hours. Once the tracheostomy is well established, care usually is given once or twice per shift, depending on the amount of drainage and secretions. Table 13-7 lists the key points in tracheostomy care.

H. Communicating with a tracheostomy patient

Communication is often quite frustrating for both the patient and the nurse. For patients on mechanical ventilators, there are talking trach tubes that allow air to flow through a tube above the cuff and over the vocal cords while keeping the cuff inflated and maintaining adequate ventilation (see Figure 13-5). You may need to experiment with various methods of communication. What works best will depend on the patient's energy level, his interest in learning new techniques, and the availability of equipment. Here are some suggestions:

TABLE 13-5

BLIND INTRATRACHEAL SUCTIONING (TRACHEAL SUCTIONING
WITHOUT USING AN ARTIFICIAL TRACHEAL AIRWAY)

Open suction catheter kit (glove, catheter, basin)

Fill basin with sterile normal saline

Squeeze water-soluble lubricant onto area of sterile field

Turn on suction source (suction pressure should not exceed
120 mm Hg)

Position patient in semi-Fowler's position (if possible) with neck slightly
hyperextended

Have patient take several deep breaths through oxygen source
(if prescribed)

Place sterile glove on dominant hand

Lubricate suction catheter with lubricant

Insert catheter through nose or mouth to the pharynx

Have patient breathe slowly and deeply as catheter is advanced
across the glottis

Evaluate placement in trachea by:

  Listening for airway sounds transmitted

  Presence of episode of coughing

  Inability to make a sound

Attach catheter to suction source and apply suction while withdrawing
and rotating catheter. Suction should not exceed 15 sec

Do not remove catheter from trachea completely, but disconnect from
suction source and have patient take several deep breaths with
oxygen

Repeat procedure until clear; then withdraw completely

Rinse catheter and tubing

Suction nasal and oropharyngeal cavity after completing intratracheal
suctioning

Discard catheter, glove, and basin

Note: Frequency of suctioning should be determined by the professional nurse.

Encourage the patient to occlude the trach tube opening
with his finger when he needs to talk (the cuff must be
deflated); offer a slate or pad and pencil; try lip reading;
or show the patient how to use an electric larynx.

I. Assessment of patient with artificial airway

You will need to assess the patient constantly for signs of
distress, hypoxia, and hypercapnia. You should also evaluate the particular artificial airway for patency and function.

TABLE 13-6

TRACHEAL SUCTIONING WITH A TRACHEOSTOMY
OR ENDOTRACHEAL TUBE

Turn on suction source (pressure should not exceed 120 mm Hg)

Open suction catheter kit (gloves, catheter, basin)

Fill basin with sterile normal saline

Place sterile glove on dominant hand

Pick up suction catheter in gloved hand and connect to suction

Instill 3 to 5 ml normal saline into tube if secretions are thick

Hyperinflate/hyperoxygenate for several deep breaths with manual
resuscitator bag (see Chapter 14)

Insert catheter as far as it will go without applying suction

Apply suction while withdrawing catheter, rotating it as you go (suction
should not exceed 15 sec)

Reoxygenate and inflate patient for several breaths

Repeat steps 8 to 10 to clear airway of secretions. Rinse catheter in
basin with sterile normal saline between suction attempts if necessary

Suction oropharyngeal cavity after completing tracheal suctioning

Discard catheter, glove, and basin

Note: Frequency of suctioning should be determined by the professional nurse.

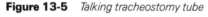

Figure 13-5 *Talking tracheostomy tube*

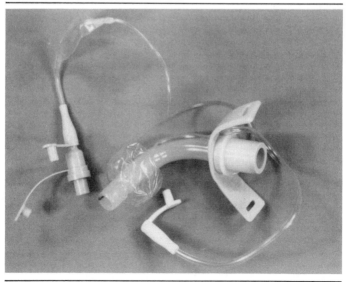

TABLE 13-7

TRACHEOSTOMY CARE

Guidelines

Use strict aseptic technique when handling anything that comes in contact with the tracheal stoma or trachea

Have a spare tracheostomy tube, a tracheostomy care kit, a suction catheter kit, and suction at the patient's bedside at all times

The professional nurse is responsible for assessing and documenting the need for and frequency of tracheostomy care

Tracheostomy care should be done approximately every 8 hours or as needed

Steps

Refer to suctioning procedure and manual resuscitator bag technique as needed

Suction tracheostomy and oropharynx

Remove soiled tracheostomy dressing

Discard dressing, glove, and catheter

Open tracheostomy care tray. Separate three basins. Pour hydrogen peroxide in one basin and sterile normal saline in another

Perform the following steps if patient has a tracheostomy tube with an inner cannula:

Remove inner cannula and immerse it in hydrogen peroxide

Suction the outer cannula

Put on sterile gloves and, using brush or pipe cleaners, clean secretions from inner cannula

Rinse inner cannula in basin with sterile normal saline

Reinsert inner cannula into tracheostomy and lock; reconnect it to ventilator or oxygen source if applicable

Clean around tracheal stoma using cotton swabs (Q-tips) or 4×4s moistened with peroxide

Follow with cotton swabs or 4×4s moistened with sterile normal saline

Inspect tracheal stoma for signs of bleeding or infection

Replace twill tape around neck with enough room to allow two fingers to slip under tape

Apply new tracheostomy dressing

Discard catheters, gloves, tracheostomy care trays, and solutions

1. Oral or nasal pharyngeal airways

Check to see whether tape, if used, is clean and secure, whether there is inflammation or excoriation in the corners of the mouth (oral) or nares (nasal), and whether there is persistent gagging (airway may be too large).

2. Endotracheal or tracheostomy tubes

Determine if there are secretions in the tube, if the tube is fastened securely and properly positioned, if there is air in the cuff and if it is properly inflated (see above for cuff inflation technique), if the humidification source is functioning properly, if there is inflammation or excoriation around the mouth or nares (endotracheal tube) or around the trach stoma (tracheostomy tube), the date of insertion or last tube change, the type and size of tube, if there is a spare tube of same size at bedside, and if the suction equipment is available and functioning. Auscultate for bilateral breath sounds and the presence of secretions in the lungs.

QUIZ

1. Match each airway with appropriate indication:

Oral airway _____

Nasal airway _____

Endotracheal tube _____

Tracheostomy tube _____

a. Used when frequent blind suctioning is required

b. Used for emergency and/or short-term intubations

c. Used to prevent patient from biting down on endotracheal tube or tongue

d. Used for patients who need prolonged ventilatory assistance

2. Indicate whether the following tube characteristics refer to endotracheal tube (ETT), tracheostomy tube (TT), or both:

Made of polyvinyl chloride and disposable _____

Can be kept in place for a prolonged period _____

Has a large, low-pressure cuff for inflation and seal _____

Requires only 1 to 2 minutes for placement _____

Equipped with a 15-mm universal adapter _____

3. List five complications that may occur in patients with long-term tracheostomy tubes:

4. The optimal cuff pressure range is between _____ and _____ cm H_2O.

5. When a cuff is inflated, an adequate seal is assessed by performing what three maneuvers?

ANSWERS

1. Oral airway **c**.

Nasal airway **a**.

Endotracheal tube **b**.

Tracheostomy tube **d**.

2. Made of polyvinyl chloride and disposable both.

Can be kept in place for a prolonged period TT.

Has a large, low-pressure cuff for inflation and seal both.

Requires only 1 to 2 minutes for placement ETT.

Equipped with a 15-mm universal adapter both.

3. Brachiocephalic trunk (innominate artery) rupture, infection, tracheoesophageal fistula, tracheal ischemia and necrosis, dysphagia, airway obstruction, tracheal dilation.

4. 15; 25.

5. Auscultating for gurgling on expiration, feeling for air leak around the nose and mouth, determining whether the patient can make a sound.

14

Respiratory Therapy Techniques

Robert J. Boyda, B.S.

OBJECTIVES

After completing this chapter, you will be able to:

1. *List the modes of oxygen therapy available to treat the hypoxic patient*

2. *Describe when IPPB, aerosol therapy, and incentive spirometry should be used for different types of patients*

3. *Demonstrate how to use chest physiotherapy (CPT) to help patients remove secretions*

4. *Demonstrate deep breathing and coughing techniques*

5. *Use a manual resuscitator bag.*

A. Oxygen therapy

The primary reason for using oxygen therapy is hypoxia, which may be caused by any number of factors (e.g., ARF, fibrosis, circulatory failure, hemorrhage, secretions in the lungs). Remember that oxygen is a drug and therefore must be ordered by a physician. Both the potential hazards (e.g., hypoventilation, oxygen toxicity, respiratory depression) and the benefits need to be recognized. Treating a patient with oxygen will alleviate the particular symptom, but the physician must treat the cause. Today there are many different oxygen devices; all will deliver oxygen if used as prescribed and if proper installation is maintained. When administering oxygen, you must pay attention to the flow rate, the oxygen percentage, and the proper connection (Table 14-1).

1. Cannulas

Prongs are the simplest of the low-flow devices and they are quite comfortable to wear. Prongs can be cut for proper placement and they can remain in position while the patient eats or takes oral medication. However, they cannot be controlled for oxygen concentration, and for prolonged use at a flow exceeding 4 liters/minute (lpm) they may cause drying and irritation of the nasal mucosa.

2. Masks

Simple masks are generally used for low- to moderate-flow oxygen, while partial or nonrebreathing masks are used for moderate- to high-flow oxygen. Although popular, these masks cannot be used for controlled oxygen concentrations and must be adjusted for proper fit. They should not press tightly against the skin and cut off circulation; adjustable elastic bands are provided to ensure comfort and security. Bags on nonrebreather masks must remain inflated during both inspiration and expiration.

Venturi masks are the most accurate and reliable. The oxygen percentages are preset and the masks can accurately deliver a known concentration at the recommended flow. As with all masks, however, they must be removed for the patient to eat or drink.

Aerosol masks, trach collars, and face tents are used with humidity devices (nebulizers) that can be adjusted for oxygen concentrations anywhere from 25 to 100 percent. If the oxygen flow falls below patient demand, room air will be pulled in. You need to make sure that a mist is constantly available for the patient during the entire inspiratory phase.

3. Other devices

Aerosol T or Briggs adapters also require a variable-oxygen-controlled nebulizer. To use such an adapter, the patient must have an endotracheal or tracheostomy tube inserted. Furthermore, excess water that accumulates in the large-bore tubing must be removed periodically or it will enter the lungs. Using a heater with these nebulizers is highly advisable, but it will increase the amount of water in the tubing. A flexible tube approximately 5 to 6 inches long on the exhalation side of the T adapter will stabilize the per-

TABLE 14-1

OXYGEN DEVICES AND SETTINGS

Device	Suggested flow rate (lpm)	O₂ percentage setting*
Cannula	1- 2	21-24*
	3- 6	24-30*
	6	35*
Mask, simple	2- 8	25-40*
	8	40-60*
Mask, partial rebreather	5- 7	30-50*
	8-12	50-75*
	12	75-95*
Mask, nonrebreather	8-12	65-80*
	12	80-100*
Mask, Venturi	4- 6	24, 26, 28
	6- 8	30, 35, 40
Mask, aerosol	4-10	30-100
Trach collar	4-10	30-100
T, Briggs	4-10	30-100
Face tent	4-10	30-100

*Settings marked with an asterisk are approximate; others are actual.

centage of oxygen being delivered. As with all aerosols, keep the mist visible to ensure proper flow.

Any oxygen device should be checked for proper delivery and accuracy, but all patients should be assessed and monitored by means of ABGs to make sure that a normal P_aO_2 is maintained for that patient (see Table 14-2).

B. IPPB therapy

IPPB is applied by a mechanical device that delivers a prescribed medication. When the patient inspires, the machine delivers an above-atmospheric-pressure breath; after the inspired air reaches a preset pressure, there is passive expiration. The IPPB machine may be powered by electricity or gas and may be connected with a mouthpiece, mask, or trach adapter.

In recent years there has been controversy over the usefulness of IPPB therapy. There is no indisputable evidence regarding its value.

1. Indications

IPPB is typically used when there are acute or chronic lung problems, in acute pulmonary edema, to assist the mobilization of secretions, in cases of drug overdose, to increase ventilation, to decrease the work of breathing, to reduce car-

TABLE 14-2

FACTORS TO WATCH FOR IN PATIENTS ON OXYGEN

Cardiac	Respiratory	Neurologic	Other
Angina	Analyze oxygen concentration	Confusion	Age (P_aO_2 decreases with age)
Cardiac output	Monitor P_aO_2	Headache	
Blood Pressure	Respiratory rate	Inappropriate behavior	Cool extremities
ECG	Dyspnea	Irritability	Cyanosis
Capillary refill	Respiratory patterns	Lethargy	Diaphoresis
Pulse	Respiratory depression	Poor concentration	Fatigue
		Restlessness	Nausea-vomiting
		Mood changes	Position (sitting for best P_aO_2)
		Coma	Skin pallor

diac output, in cases of restrictive lung impairments, for sputum induction, and to prevent or treat postoperative atelectasis. Its primary function, however, is to deliver medications deep in the lower respiratory tract.

2. Hazards

IPPB can cause pneumothorax, mucosal drying, increased intracranial pressure, hemoptysis, gastric insufflation, vomiting with possible aspiration, dependency (with long-term use, as in COPD), hyperventilation, excessive oxygen (due to uncontrolled oxygen-air dilution), or cardiovascular or circulatory problems.

3. Considerations

In order to use IPPB properly, it is important to instruct the patient correctly during his initial treatment; make sure the patient is coherent, cooperative, and relaxed; see that the patient is not exhausted and is positioned properly (as upright as possible); monitor volume (exhaled V_T must be above the normal V_T) and improved peak flow rates; encourage the patient to cough after each treatment; and assess the patient afterward (note amount, consistency, and color of sputum).

C. Hand-held aerosol/mini-nebulizer therapy

This apparatus disperses a liquid (medication) into microscopic particles and delivers it to the lungs by the air movement of the patient's breath. The mini-nebulizer is usually air-driven by means of a compressor* via connecting tubing; however, in some instances where the patient can tolerate oxygen, he may be treated via a flowmeter and nipple at a rate of 3 to 6 lpm. As with any type of aerosol-generating apparatus, a mist must be visible and available for the patient to inhale.

1. Indications

These are similar to the indications for IPPB except that the patient must be cooperative since he must generate a larger

---

*A hand-squeezed, bulb-type nebulizer can be used, but first you should assess the patient's energy level for this work.

than normal breath without the aid of the positive pressure machine. Diaphragmatic breathing is helpful as a technique for proper use of the mini-nebulizer.

2. Hazards

The hazards of mini-nebulizer treatment are essentially those of IPPB.

3. Considerations

In addition to the factors listed for the proper use of IPPB, the patient should breathe through his mouth, take slow, deep breaths, and hold his breath for a few seconds at the end of inspiration (to increase intrapleural pressure and recruit collapsed alveoli, thereby increasing FRC). You should encourage the patient to cough and assess his progress with the therapy.

D. Incentive spirometry

With this technique, a mechanical device provides the patient with goal-oriented maneuvers to increase ventilation. Disposable incentive spirometers utilize a ball or disk in a tube (flow) or an accordion/bellows (volume) mechanism. There are also electronic types with visual displays. Most electronic and some disposable spirometers can also record and display the number of goals set and the number of goals achieved.

TABLE 14-3

ASSESSMENT OF PATIENTS FOR CPT

Cardiac	*Physical*	*Respiratory*	*Other*
Blood pressure	Current status	Arterial blood gases	Emotional/ mental status
Cardiac output	Pain	Breath sounds	IPPB or nebulizer therapy
Cardiopathy	Prognosis	Chest X-ray	Nursing goals
ECG	Restrictions or limitations	Pulmonary function studies	Physician's order
Positional hypotension	Untreated conditions	Sputum production	Overall treatment plan

1. Indications

Incentive spirometers are used preoperatively to maintain normal lung function and postoperatively to prevent or treat atelectasis, hypoxia, hypercapnia, and shunting. In other cases, the physician should document the medical necessity for incentive spirometry.

As prophylaxis, spirometry is more effective than the overutilized IPPB since it is less costly and requires less personnel time.

2. Hazards

The only hazard is hypoventilation and its effects.

3. Considerations

For incentive spirometry, it is important to make sure that the patient is coherent, cooperative, and relaxed; instruct him as to the reason for this therapy; make sure he is as erect as possible; teach him diaphragmatic breathing (slow, constant inspiration); instruct him to hold his breath at the end of inspiration (at least 3 seconds) and to exhale slowly and completely; teach him to cough during and after session; help splint the patient's incision site; set a reasonable goal (in order not to discourage the patient); have spirometry device within the patient's reach; start therapy immediately postoperatively (atelectasis starts 1 hour after hypoventilation begins); make sure the patient does not try to exceed his set goals or his tolerance; and, every 1 to 2 hours, assess treatment and record the number of goals achieved.

E. Chest physiotherapy

This is the application of specific physical exercises to improve lung function. Prior to CPT, the patient is assessed to devise an individually tailored plan (Table 14-3).

1. Types

a. Postural drainage. This is the positioning of a patient to take advantage of gravity as an aid in removing retained secretions from lung segments (see Table 14-4). A bed or flat table should be utilized.

TABLE 14-4

POSTURAL DRAINAGE

Segmental bronchi	Patient's postural position	Area for percussion/vibration
Right and left upper lobes		
Apical segment	Lying back, head raised to 30° angle	Over area between clavicle and top of scapula
Anterior segment	Lying flat, pillow under knees	Between clavicle and nipple
Posterior segment	Sitting up, leaning forward against pillow on abdominal area	Upper third of back over ribs
Left lingula		
Inferior-superior	Head down on right side; rotate ¼ turn back; support with pillow; knees flexed	Left nipple area
Right middle lobe		
Lateral medial	Head down on left side; rotate ¼ turn back; support with pillow; knees flexed	Right nipple area
Left and right lower lobes		
Anterior basal	Head down on side; arm raised over head; pillow under knees; or—head down lying on back	Lower ribs just beneath axilla
Lateral basal	Head down on abdomen; rotate ¼ turn up; upper leg flexed	Middle third of ribs
Posterior basal	Head down flat on abdomen, pillow under hips	Lower third of ribs
Superior segment	Lying flat on abdomen, pillow under hips	Middle of third ribs on back from tip of scapula on either side of spine

How long a patient should remain in a given position will depend upon his tolerance. Ideally, positions should be maintained for 15 to 20 minutes, concentrating on the involved areas.

b. Percussion. Chest percussion is performed by cupping or clapping the chest wall (by creating an air pocket with the hand) in a rhythmical fashion. When done over the involved segment (together with postural drainage), percussion can dislodge mucus plugs and allow air to push them up the bronchial tree. Percussion ought to be maintained for about 3 to 5 minutes, alternating with vibration. The patient should then be allowed to rest while taking in deep breaths through his mouth and exhaling through pursed lips. He should attempt a few coughs and then the entire procedure needs to be repeated.

Be sure to use a thin sheet or towel to protect the patient's skin during percussion. Check the skin to make sure that there is no redness; the force of percussion should never hurt the patient.

c. Vibration. This technique increases the velocity of exhaled air and can help eliminate the secretions being drained. Chest vibration is performed by laying one hand flat on top of the other over an involved area. The hands are then rapidly vibrated.

Vibration should be done only on exhalation and can be performed together with percussion and deep breathing. Because vibration requires the performer to expend a lot of energy, a mechanical vibrator may be substituted.

2. Indications

CPT is frequently used before and after abdominal and thoracic surgery; for breathing retraining; for ventilator patients; and for patients with atelectasis, COPD, ineffective cough, neuromuscular disorders, and restrictive lung disease.

3. Hazards

Some of the problems encountered with CPT include dyspnea, fatigue, fractured ribs, increased pain, increased bronchospasms in asthmatics, increased pulmonic bleeding, increased venous return on postural drainage, and the spread of infections or tumors.

4. Considerations

With CPT it is important to make sure that the patient is comfortable and not wearing restrictive clothing. Start with the uppermost area and proceed to lower areas. Give medication for pain before CPT, splint the incision, and use pillow support. Vary positions, but focus on the affected area. Return the patient to a comfortable position; never leave him in a position he cannot get out of. Discontinue therapy if the patient has normal respirations, can mobilize secretions, has clear chest X-ray, and has normal breath sounds.

F. Deep breathing

This may be used for breathing retraining or as an adjunct to CPT. Whenever teaching any of these techniques to a patient, always make sure he is comfortable; start slowly and easily, progressing further each time without exhausting him. Exhalation should take approximately twice as long as inspiration. These exercises will improve ventilation and decrease oxygen consumption, but more important, they will give the patient proper control and enable him to use his available energy efficiently for breathing.

1. Diaphragmatic breathing

This technique will decrease the use of accessory neck muscles and will help strengthen the diaphragm. First, instruct the patient to sit in a relaxed position (after mastering the technique, the patient can do it while standing or walking). Place one hand on the upper chest and one on the abdomen. Have the patient exhale; at the same time, your hand should gently push his abdomen in. On inhalation, his abdomen should push your hand out. Repeat 10 to 20 times. While the patient is exhaling, it is helpful if he uses pursed lip breathing (especially if he is dyspneic).

Weights of 2 to 5 pounds can be used instead of hands since the diaphragm is a muscle. Eventually the patient will be able to do this exercise without using either hands or weights.

2. Pursed lip breathing

With this technique, the patient should first take in a normal breath slowly through the nose. He should then purse his lips (like blowing through a straw) and exhale slowly.

Have him repeat this several times in conjunction with diaphragmatic breathing. The patient might practice by blowing against the flame of a candle without blowing it out. Move the candle away little by little until the flame does not waver. Then have the patient practice blowing it out from this distance.

3. Segmental breathing

This technique is difficult and focuses on an area where increased muscular effort and expansion are needed. It is done by placing your hand over the affected area (segment); with a slight pressure from your hand and with the patient using pursed lips, instruct him to move that particular area by exhaling.

4. Coughing

Coughing (or the rapid expulsion of air) is a protective mechanism produced by stimulation of the larynx, trachea, and larger bronchi. The technique for coughing is as follows: While he is sitting, have the patient breathe in and hold it. Ask him to contract his abdominal and throat muscles. Then, instruct him to exhale forcefully three or more short (staccato) coughs. You may support the patient by putting your hands on the lower part of the chest over the diaphragm and pushing gently during exhalation. Repeat. Intubated patients can be helped to cough by lavaging a small amount of saline solution and bagging several times. Follow this with suctioning. Postoperative patients can be given pain medications before coughing. Teach them how to splint the incision by using pillows.

G. Manual ventilation (bagging)

Manual resuscitators are compliant, self-inflating bags that deliver positive pressure on compression. They also contain a nonrebreathing valve that supplies air or oxygen to the patient and allows inspiration to take place. On exhalation, the valve allows air to go around it and out the exhalation port to the surrounding atmosphere. The patient is ventilated through a mask or tracheostomy or endotracheal tube connection. An oxygen reservoir may be added to enrich the air delivered to the patient via the bag.

1. Indications

Manual resuscitators are used to ventilate patients during CPR; to provide manual hyperinflation at high levels of oxygen before, during, and after suctioning of the airway, and to provide or assist ventilation for apneic or ventilator-dependent patients en route from one area to another.

2. Hazards

Potential hazards include gastric insufflation or vomiting due to poor technique, hyperventilation, pneumothorax, and infection as a result of equipment contamination.

3. Technique

Place an airway in the patient if he doesn't already have a tracheostomy or endotracheal tube. If you're using a mask, grasp the patient's chin, place the rounded part of the mask on his chin under the lower lip, and apply the narrow part to the bridge of his nose and tight against his cheeks. With the same hand holding the patient's chin, tilt his head back. Squeeze the bag quickly and firmly with the other hand (its maximum volume is 1 liter). Watch for chest excursion. Release the bag to permit exhalation.

Keep the respiratory rate between 12 and 20/minute. During CPR, keep the rate at one per every five chest compressions. Continue to assist breathing until the patient's effort or respiration returns to normal (or he is placed on a ventilator).

4. Considerations

When using a manual resuscitator, be sure to test the bag by squeezing it and observing if it is in proper working order. Always keep the unit assembled (mask attached) and ready for use. When using with artificial airway, keep the mask available in case of inadvertent decannulation or extubation. Keep the flow rate high enough to entrain oxygen during inhalation (set the flow rate at 10 to 15 lpm).

Use an oxygen reservoir when available (up to 50 percent oxygen without reservoir and up to 95 percent oxygen with reservoir). Allow more time for exhalation than inspiration (a longer inflation time allows more O_2 to enter). Clean and sterilize bags and masks after each use. Change bags routinely (perhaps every 24 hours) for tracheostomy or endotracheal tube patient.

QUIZ

1. Which of the following is *not* an important consideration in order for patient to receive proper breathing treatment with IPPB, aerosol therapy, or incentive spirometry?

   a. Patient should be instructed properly.

   b. Patient should not be allowed to cough during treatment.

   c. Patient should be assessed for the effect of each treatment.

   d. Patient should be sitting upright as much as possible.

2. True or false:

   There is controversy regarding the usefulness of IPPB _____

   An aerosol nebulizer delivers microscopic particles of liquid (medication) to the lungs _____

   Incentive spirometry is goal-oriented deep breathing designed to improve ventilation _____

3. Postural drainage is the positioning of a patient to utilize _____ to aid in secretion removal.

4. The effectiveness of CPT can be determined by evaluating the following three factors:

5. The most effective muscle of breathing is the

_____ .

6. To provide for hyperinflation before, during, and after suctioning, what apparatus is used?

7. Match the mode of oxygen therapy with the correct oxygen percentage range:

Nasal cannula _____   **a.** 24, 26, 28, 30, 35, 40%

Partial rebreather mask _____   **b.** 65-100%

Nonrebreather mask _____   **c.** 21-35%

Venturi _____   **d.** 30-95%

ANSWERS

1. **b.**
2. True.
   True.
   True.
3. Gravity.
4. Blood gases, breath sounds, sputum production (see Table 14-2 for more).
5. Diaphragm.
6. Manual resuscitator bag.
7. Nasal cannula **c.**
   Partial rebreather mask **d.**
   Nonrebreather mask **b.**
   Venturi **a.**

15

Mechanical Ventilation

OBJECTIVES

After completing this chapter, you will be able to:

1. List the major classifications of ventilators and explain the use of each

2. Assess the ventilatory status of a patient on a mechanical ventilator

3. Evaluate the status of a volume ventilator attached to a patient

4. List four potential problems associated with mechanical ventilation.

A. Indications for using mechanical ventilators

If a patient is experiencing increasing respiratory failure due to a thoracotomy or upper abdominal incision, drug overdose, neuromuscular disease, inhalation injury, acute respiratory infection superimposed on COPD, multiple trauma and shock, multisystem failure, or unconsciousness, mechanical ventilation may be necessary. However, the decision to place the patient on a ventilator should be determined by the presence of apnea, a P_aO_2 of less than 50 mm Hg with supplemental oxygen, a P_aCO_2 of more than 50 mm Hg causing acidosis, and/or a respiratory rate of more than 35 (see Table 15-1).

B. Classification

1. Negative pressure

These ventilators exert a negative pressure on the external chest, thereby causing it and the underlying lung to expand. Although they were quite common many years ago when polio was prevalent, they are not used much now in the acute care setting. Examples include the iron lung and the portable chest cuirass ventilator.

2. Positive pressure

These are the most commonly used ventilators today. They inflate the lungs by exerting positive pressure on the airway, forcing the alveoli to expand. For long-term use, intubation or tracheostomy is necessary. There are two main types.

a. Pressure-cycled ventilators. With this type, we determine and control the positive inspiratory pressure reached with each breath. In other words, the machine cycles on, delivering air (and oxygen) until a certain pressure is reached, then it cycles off. The disadvantage is that you cannot be sure about the volume of air or oxygen delivered with each breath, so a patient with increased airway resistance or decreased compliance may not get enough air. Furthermore, these machines have no alarms, sighs (see below), or source of humidification. They are intended for short-term use only,

TABLE 15-1

CRITERIA FOR MECHANICAL VENTILATION

$P_aO_2 < 50$ mm Hg with $F_iO_2 > 0.60$
$P_aCO_2 > 50$ mm Hg with pH < 7.25
$VC < 2 \times V_T$
Negative inspiratory force < 25 cm H_2O
$RR > 35$

such as for IPPB treatment or postoperatively in the recovery room.

b. Volume-cycled ventilators. With this type, we determine the volume of air to be delivered with each breath. From breath to breath, the patient can be assured of receiving an appropriate volume for adequate ventilation. Volume-cycled ventilators are intended for long-term use, for patients with primary pulmonary disease, or for patients with an impaired bellows mechanism (neuromuscular disease). The models commonly seen in the acute care setting include Bennett MA-1 and MA-2+2, Bear 1 and 2, Ohio 560, Servo, and Engstrom.

c. Time-cycled ventilators. These ventilators terminate inspiration after a preset time. Tidal volume is regulated by adjusting the length of inspiration and the flow rate. This type is appropriate for neonates and infants, but is rarely used for adults.

C. Functions and settings of volume ventilators

1. Tidal volume

This is the amount of air exchanged with each breath. When a patient is on a ventilator, this should be about 10 to 15 ml/kg of body weight.

2. Respiratory rate

The respiratory rate is usually set between 10 and 16 breaths per minute.

3. Oxygen concentration

The percentage of oxygen used will vary according to the patient's condition. The volume ventilator can deliver between 21 and 100 percent oxygen.

4. Pressure

Volume-cycled ventilators have an upper-limit setting, which is the greatest pressure the ventilator will use to push in the air. However, the actual airway pressure varies from breath to breath in order to assure an adequate tidal volume. The upper limit is usually set from 15 to 20 cm H_2O above the normal inspiratory pressure.

5. Flow rate

This is the speed at which the air is delivered. It determines inspiratory time and is usually 40 to 60 lpm for adults.

6. Modes for controlling ventilation

There are several ways in which ventilation is controlled mechanically:

a. Controlled mechanical ventilation. The machine delivers a set number of breaths and ignores any inspiratory effort.

b. Assist/control ventilation. The machine is sensitive to the patient's negative inspiratory effort. It delivers the preset tidal volume whenever the patient's effort is strong enough to trigger the ventilator. If the patient fails to take a breath within the allotted time, the machine will deliver a controlled breath to the patient.

c. Intermittent mandatory ventilation. The machine is set to deliver a certain number of breaths per minute. Between those breaths, the patient may take spontaneous breaths of whatever tidal volume he is capable of. These breaths are humidified and oxygenated just like the mandatory breaths. The number of mandatory breaths can gradually be reduced on the machine. Consequently, intermittent mandatory ventilation (IMV) is helpful in weaning the patient from the ventilator.

d. Synchronized IMV. This is similar to IMV except that when the mandatory breath is due, it is delivered in conjunction with the next spontaneous inspiratory effort. This method is supposed to be a more comfortable one for the patient.

7. Sighs

A normal sigh provides a periodic deep breath that inflates more alveoli, thereby preventing atelectasis, and also stimulates surfactant production. The ventilator can also produce sighs once we set the volume (200 ml to twice the tidal volume), rate (8 to 10 sighs/hour), and pressure limit (15 to 20 cm H_2O above the normal inspiratory pressure).

8. Alarms

Ventilators have a variety of alarms to help you monitor your patient's status. Alarms indicate low volume, high pressure, low pressure, temperature of humidification sources, inappropriate inspiratory to expiratory ratios, and PEEP levels.

9. PEEP/CPAP

Most volume ventilators provide PEEP, which is used to keep alveoli open during expiration, thereby enhancing oxygenation and allowing lower concentrations of oxygen to be delivered. Continuous positive airway pressure (CPAP) achieves the same thing in the alveoli as PEEP, but it does so in the spontaneously breathing patient.

D. Problems with mechanical ventilation

Because of the highly complex and technical nature of mechanical ventilation and the seriousness of the patient's condition, a number of problems can arise: inadequate alveolar ventilation; an air leak in the system; a cuff leak; obstruction or resistance to air flow; too much condensation in the tubing; bucking the ventilator (when the patient fights the machine); secretions, bronchospasm, decreased compliance; atelectasis; respiratory alkalosis (from overventilation on the machine); propensity to ulcer disease; decreased venous return; and the inability to communicate.

E. Assessment of the patient and machine

It is important to make sure the patient is receiving adequate ventilation and oxygenation. Check the following: vital signs; evidence of hypoxia; respiratory rate and pattern; breath sounds; neurologic status; tidal volume, minute ventilation, and forced vital capacity; nutritional state; suctioning needs; psychological state (patient's readiness to be weaned); patient's inspiratory effort; and bucking the ventilator.

The ventilator also needs to be assessed to make sure that it is functioning properly and that the settings are appropriate. You should note the type of machine, the mode of controlling ventilation, the settings for tidal volume and respiratory rate, the F_iO_2, the inspiratory pressure and the upper-limit setting, whether the sigh setting is on or off, whether there is water in the tubing, whether the humidifier is filled, whether the alarms have been properly set, the PEEP level (if used), and whether the tubing is kinked or disconnected.

QUIZ

1. Pressure-cycled ventilators (do/do not) control volume delivered, and so they are for short-term use only.

Since volume-cycled ventilators deliver a preset _____ , they can assure adequate ventilation.

2. List four factors that should be assessed in the patient on a ventilator:

3. List four factors that should be assessed to make sure that the ventilator is functioning properly:

4. List four potential problems associated with mechanical ventilation:

1. Do not; volume.

2. Tidal volume, minute ventilation, FVC; breath sounds; evidence of hypoxia; patient compliance; vital signs; respiratory rate and pattern; neurologic status; nutritional state; suctioning needs; readiness to be weaned.

3. Type of machine, F_iO_2 setting, ventilator mode, water in tubing, sigh setting on or off, settings for tidal volume and respiratory rate, inspiratory pressure, upper-limit setting, humidifier filled, alarms set, PEEP level, tubing kinked or disconnected.

4. Inadequate alveolar ventilation, increased ulcer disease, inability to communicate, too much condensation in tubing, air leak, cuff leak, obstruction or resistance to air flow, secretions, bronchospasm, decreased compliance, atelectasis, respiratory alkalosis due to overventilation, decreased venous return.

GLOSSARY

Acidosis — a low blood pH level (below 7.35) caused by excessive acid or loss of base

Adenoma — a neoplasm of glandular epithelium

Aerobic metabolism — cell functions that take place only in the presence of oxygen

Alkalosis — a high blood pH level (above 7.45) caused by excessive accumulation of base or loss of acid

Alpha$_1$-antitrypsin — a serum protein that inhibits the formation of elastase; a deficiency of this protein causes emphysema

Anaerobic metabolism — cell functions that take place only in the absence of oxygen

Angle of Louis — the fissure between the manubrium and the main body of the sternum; serves as a reference point for venous distention and level of carina

Asterixis — jerky dorsiflexion of hand when pressed and released (commonly called liver flap)

Bleb — a collection of air just beneath the pleura; caused by alveoli that rupture from overdistention

Bronchophony — clear and distinct voice sound heard through the chest; occurs in areas of consolidation

Buffer — a compound that minimizes the change in pH when an acid or a base is added

Bulla — air space within the lung tissue caused by alveolar wall destruction and overdistention and formed from many alveoli

Cardiac output — the amount of blood pumped by the heart, measured in liters per minute

Carina — the place where the right and left mainstem bronchi branch from the trachea

Cilia — hairlike projections that line the conducting airways to mobilize mucus and foreign matter upward

Compliance — the lung's ability to yield elastically when a force is applied; a measure of its distensibility, expressed as change in volume divided by change in pressure

Continuous positive airway pressure (CPAP) — provision of distending airway pressure on expiration to keep alveoli open in the spontaneously breathing patient

Cor pulmonale — right ventricular failure secondary to pulmonary disease (COPD, pulmonary hypertension, etc.)

Cyanosis — blueness of skin or mucous membranes; a late sign of hypoxia. Central cyanosis is due to decreased oxygen tension in the arterial blood; peripheral cyanosis, to decreased local supply of oxygen, e.g., fingers, legs, etc. (not life-threatening)

Dead space ventilation (V_D) — area in lung where ventilation exceeds blood flow

Diffusion — movement of a substance (gas) from an area of greater concentration to an area of lesser concentration

Egophony — the sound heard when a patient says "E" but as it comes through the chest wall it changes to "A"; occurs in pleural effusion, abscess, and consolidation

Fenestration — an opening or window (in tracheostomy tubes it is a means to encourage use of the upper airway)

Fibrosis — formation of abnormal tissue that contains fibers; causes scarring and stiffening in the lung

Fraction of inspired oxygen (F_iO_2) — the fraction of inhaled air that is oxygen (expressed as a decimal)

Fremitus — palpable respiratory vibrations felt with or without vocalization

Functional residual capacity (FRC) — the volume of air in the lungs at the end of normal expiration

Hypoventilation (alveolar) — inadequate ventilation at the alveolar level; occurs when P_aCO_2 is above 45 mm Hg

Hypoxemia (decreased P_aO_2) — decreased oxygen tension in the arterial blood (below 80 mm Hg)

Hypoxia — decreased oxygen supply to the tissues

Intermittent mandatory ventilation (IMV) — a form of mechanical ventilation in which ventilator breathing is interspersed between the patient's spontaneous breaths

Intrapulmonary shunting — a diversion in which some of the blood going through the lungs returns to the heart unoxygenated

Minute ventilation ($\dot{V}_E$) – the volume of air breathed in 1 minute (tidal volume times rate)

Mucosal hyperplasia – formation of excessive mucous membranes

Negative inspiratory force (NIF) – negative pressure generated at the beginning of inspiration; measures muscle strength for breathing

Oxygenation – the process of gas exchange in which oxygen diffuses from the alveoli into the capillaries and then to tissue cells

Oxygen consumption (VO_2) – volume of oxygen consumed by the body in 1 minute

Oxygen saturation – the percentage of total hemoglobin that is saturated with oxygen

Oxyhemoglobin – the combined form of hemoglobin and oxygen

Papilledema – edema and inflammation of the optic nerve at its entrance to the eyeball

Paradoxical breathing – breathing in which the chest wall deflates during inspiration and inflates during expiration instead of the reverse

Partial pressure – pressure exerted by each component of a mixture of gases

Pectus carinatum – abnormal prominence of the sternum

Pectus excavatum – congenital condition in which the sternum is abnormally depressed

Perfusion ($\dot{Q}$) – the volume of blood per unit of time flowing through a vascular bed (in the lungs it is the pulmonary circulation)

pH – symbol indicating hydrogen ion concentration; pH above 7 is alkaline and pH below 7 is acid

Phagocytosis – ingestion of bacteria and other foreign particles by phagocytes

Pores of Kohn – tiny openings between neighboring alveoli that permit a more even distribution of air

Positive end-expiratory pressure (PEEP) – mechanical ventilation with positive pressure at the end of expiration; it is used to keep alveoli from collapsing

Rales — discontinuous, popping, crackling sounds heard mainly on inspiration and caused by air moving through liquid

Resistance — the change in pressure of a gas as it moves from an area of higher pressure to one of lower pressure divided by the rate at which the volume of gas is displaced (flow)

Respiration — the process of oxygen and carbon dioxide exchange in the lungs and at the cellular level

Rhonchi — gurgling, snoring, or moaning sounds heard mainly on expiration and caused by air moving through narrowed airways or secretion-filled airways

Sputum — substance expectorated; it contains saliva, mucus, and sometimes pus

Surfactant — a lipoprotein coating that reduces the surface tension of the alveoli, thus helping to maintain expansion

Tidal volume (V_T) — volume of air breathed in a normal inhalation or exhalation

Venous admixture — a ventilation/perfusion abnormality in which perfusion exceeds ventilation

Ventilation — the mechanical process of getting air in and out of the lungs

Vital capacity (VC) — the maximum volume of air that can be exhaled after maximum inspiration

$\dot{V}/\dot{Q}$ (ventilation/perfusion) — the relationship between alveolar ventilation and pulmonary blood flow; mismatching is a major cause of pulmonary disease

Wheezes — high-pitched, musical rhonchi heard mainly on expiration and caused by narrowing of the small airways (as in asthma)

Whispered pectoriloquy — the same voice sound as heard in bronchophony, but here the words are whispered; this is a more sensitive sound

ADDITIONAL TEST QUESTIONS

1. The only complete cartilaginous ring in the trachea is the _____ .

2. The _____ mainstem bronchus is more likely to be cannulated during endotracheal intubation because of its close alignment with the trachea.

3. The average amount of anatomical dead space in the adult is _____ ml.

4. Which alveolar cell secretes surfactant: type I, type II, or type III?

5. The three major muscle groups used in normal breathing are _____ , _____ , and _____ .

6. List two conditions in which lung compliance is decreased and the lungs are stiff:

7. Minute ventilation is a measure of _____ _____ times _____ in 1 minute.

8. The lung is ideal for the diffusion process because if the alveoli were spread out side by side, the lung would be the size of a _____ .

9. If the F_iO_2 is increased, the P_AO_2 will (increase/decrease/remain the same).

10. The relationship between oxygen tensions and hemoglobin saturation is illustrated by the _____ _____ .

11. The respiratory centers in the brain are located in the _____ and _____ .

12. List two abnormalities of the chest wall that suggest underlying lung impairment:

13. In order for cyanosis to occur as a sign of hypoxia, the amount of unoxygenated hemoglobin must be greater than _____ .

14. The act of striking the surface of the chest to elicit a sound so the underlying tissue can be evaluated is _____ .

15. The negative logarithm of hydrogen ion concentration is _____ .

16. The four buffer systems in the body are:

17. If a patient's arterial blood gases are: pH 7.49, P_aCO_2 30 mm Hg, P_aO_2 85 mm Hg, HCO_3^- 26, what is the acid-base disturbance?

18. A diagnosis of chronic bronchitis is made if the individual has a chronic cough with expectoration that lasts at least _____ months a year for _____ consecutive years.

19. A rare familial emphysema is caused by a deficiency in _____ .

20. The pulmonary function test of a patient with emphysema would show an (increased/normal/decreased) forced expiratory volume in 1 second (FEV_1).

21. Identify the type of blood gas changes that occur in a patient with severe COPD with a compensated acidosis (draw directional arrows):

pH P_aO_2
P_aCO_2 HCO_3^-

22. The incidence of postoperative pulmonary complications is greatest in the patient who has (lower abdominal surgery/local anesthesia/a smoking history).

23. List two risk factors for deep vein thrombosis:

24. Pneumonia is the _____-ranking cause of death in the United States.

25. A localized, pus-filled, necrotic lesion in the lung is called a _____ .

26. Most primary tumors in the lung arise from the bronchial epithelium and are called _____ _____ .

27. The cancer that is the leading cause of death among men in the United States is _____ .

28. The injury in which more than one rib is fractured in more than one place is called _____ _____ .

29. Venous admixture occurs in the patient with ARF or ARDS and results in _____ .

30. The edema that occurs in ARDS is called _____ _____ edema.

31. Two methods of communicating with a patient who has a tracheostomy tube are:

32. When rhonchi are heard in the right posterior base of the lung, what position should the patient be placed in for effective postural drainage?

33. The tidal volume needed for a patient on a volume ventilator is _____ ml/kg of body weight.

34. When a patient receives mechanical breaths interspersed with his own spontaneous breaths, this is called _____ .

35. The pressure in the pleural cavity of a normal intact lung is always (positive/negative).

36. The pulmonary circulation is a (low/high) pressure system.

37. When perfusion is in excess of ventilation, _____ is the result.

38. The amount of blood pumped by the heart in 1 minute is called _____ .

39. A patient is said to have labored respirations if he is using his _____ for breathing.

40. The voice sound heard over areas of the lung where the alveoli are filled with or replaced by solid tissue is called _____ .

ANSWERS

  1. Cricoid.

  2. Right. .

  3. 150 ml.

  4. Type II.

  5. Diaphragm, intercostals, abdominal.

  6. Pulmonary edema, fibrosis, abdominal distention, ARDS.

  7. Tidal volume; rate.

  8. Tennis court.

  9. Increase.

  10. Oxyhemoglobin dissociation curve.

  11. Pons; medulla.

  12. Increased A-P diameter, pectus excavatum, pectus carinatum, scars, kyphosis, scoliosis.

  13. 5 gm/100 ml.

  14. Percussion.

15. pH.

16. Bicarbonate ion/carbonic acid, phosphates, hemoglobin, protein.

17. Respiratory alkalosis.

18. 3; 2.

19. Alpha$_1$-antitrypsin.

20. Decreased.

21. pH↓ or normal, P_aCO_2↑, P_aO_2↓, HCO_3^- ↑.

22. A smoking history.

23. Immobility, recent surgery, obesity, age, pregnancy, trauma to legs, oral contraceptives, pre-existing lung or heart disease.

24. Fifth.

25. Lung abscess.

26. Bronchogenic carcinoma.

27. Lung cancer.

28. Flail chest.

29. Hypoxemia.

30. Noncardiogenic.

31. Finger over trach with cuff deflated, slate, pad and pencil, lip reading, electric larynx.

32. On left side, with head down and pillow under hips.

33. 10 to 15.

34. Intermittent mandatory ventilation (IMV).

35. Negative.

36. Low.

37. Venous admixture.

38. Cardiac output.

39. Accessory muscles.

40. Bronchophony.

SELECTED READINGS

Books

Anderson JM: *Occupational Lung Disease — An Introduction.* New York: American Lung Association, 1979

Armstrong ME, et al, eds: *McGraw-Hill Handbook of Clinical Nursing.* New York: McGraw-Hill, 1979

Borg N, et al: *Core Curriculum for Critical Care Nursing,* 2nd ed. Philadelphia: Saunders, 1981

Brunner LS, Suddarth DS: *Textbook of Medical-Surgical Nursing,* 4th ed. Philadelphia: Lippincott, 1980

Burton G, et al: *Respiratory Care. A Guide to Clinical Practice.* Philadelphia: Lippincott, 1977

Cherniack RM, et al: *Respiration in Health and Disease,* 2nd ed. Philadelphia: Saunders, 1972

Glennon SA, et al: *AACN Clinical Reference,* ch 23. New York: McGraw-Hill, 1980

Guyton AC: *Textbook of Medical Physiology,* 6th ed. Philadelphia: Saunders, 1981

Harper RW: *A Guide to Respiratory Care.* Philadelphia: Lippincott, 1981

Luckman J, Sorensen KC: *Medical-Surgical Nursing — A Psychophysiologic Approach,* 2nd ed. Philadelphia: Saunders, 1980

Martz KV, et al: *Management of the Patient-Ventilator System.* St. Louis: Mosby, 1979

Sharpiro BA, et al: *Clinical Application of Respiratory Care,* 3rd ed. Chicago: Year Book Medical Publishers, 1977

Periodicals

Albanese AJ, Toplitz, AD: A hassle-free guide to suctioning a tracheostomy. *RN* p 82, April 1982

ATS guidelines for use of IPPB. *Respir Care* 25:365, 1980

Benjamin SP, McCormack LJ: Structural Abnormalities in COPD. *Postgrad Med* 62:101, 1977

Boyer MW: Treating invasive lung cancer. *Am J Nurs* 77(12): 1916, 1977

Cline BA, Fisher ML: A.R.D.S. means emergency. *Nursing 82,* p 63, February 1982

Fuchs PL: Understanding continuous mechanical ventilation. *Nursing 79,* p 26, December 1979

Golish JA, Ahmad M: Management of COPD, a physiologic approach. *Postgrad Med* 62:131, 1977

Hopewell PC: Adult respiratory distress syndrome. *Basics of RD, ATS News,* p 16, summer 1979

Mitman LM: Pulmonary hypertension. *Nursing 82,* p 61, February 1982

Nielsen L: Mechanical ventilation: Patient assessment and nursing care. *Am J Nurs* 80(12): 2191, 1980

Standards for nursing care of patients with COPD. *Basics of RD, ATS News,* p 31, summer 1981

INDEX

A

Abdominal distention, 10
Abdominal muscles
  anatomy of, 8
  inspection, 37
Abdominal surgery, 85
Abnormal breath sounds, 48
Abscess (lung), 115, 118
Absent breath sounds, 48
Accessory muscles
  anatomy and, 8
  inspection and, 37
Acetylcysteine, 78
Acid-base balance
  disturbances, 62
  arterial blood gas
    interpretation, 58-64
  chronic obstructive pulmonary
    disease, 72
  compensation for, 63
  pulmonary hypertension and,
    109
Acidosis. See Metabolic
  acidosis; Respiratory acidosis
Acute respiratory failure (ARF),
  138-141
  adult respiratory distress
    syndrome and, 141
  chronic obstructive pulmonary
    disease and, 76
  etiology, 138-139
  management, 147
  occupational lung disease and,
    100
  treatment, 140-141
Adam's apple. See Thyroid cartilage
Adenocarcinoma, 126
Adenoids, 2
Adenoma (benign bronchial), 126
Adipose tissue, 48
Adrenal glands, 126
Adult respiratory distress
  syndrome (ARDS), 141-147
  acute respiratory failure and, 138
  assessment, 52-53, 143-145
  auscultation, 48

  hypoxemia and, 18
  lung contusion and, 133
  management, 147
  pathophysiology of, 142-143
  restrictive lung disease and, 84, 86
  treatment, 145-147
Adventitious breath sounds, 48-49
Aerosol masks, 167
Aerosol/mini-nebulizer therapy,
  hand-held, 169-170
Aerosol T adapters, 167
Age. See also Elderly
  emphysema and, 73
  inspection and, 34-35
Air pollution
  chronic obstructive pulmonary
    disease and, 73
  occupational lung disease, 90
  patient history and, 26-27
  pulmonary tumors and, 127
Air pressure, 9
Airway
  adult respiratory distress
    syndrome and, 147
  anatomy, 2-4
  blood supply, 8-9
  chest trauma and, 130
  rhonchi, 48-49
  wheezes, 49
Airway management, 150-163
  chronic obstructive pulmonary
    disease and, 77-78
  endotracheal tubes, 151-153
  manual ventilation, 176
  nasopharyngeal airway, 150-151
  oropharyngeal airway, 150
  tracheostomy tubes, 153-162
Airway obstruction
  chest trauma, 130
  chronic obstructive pulmonary
    disease, 74
Airway resistance, 10-11, 70
Albuterol, 77
Alkalosis. See Metabolic alkalosis;
  Respiratory alkalosis
  medical correction of, 64

Allergic alveolitis, 91, 94-95
Allergy
    asthma and, 71
    chronic obstructive pulmonary
        disease and, 73
    patient history, 26-27
    pulmonary fibrosis and, 86
Alpha$_1$-antitrypsin
    emphysema and, 73
    patient history and, 26
Alveolar-capillary network, 8, 11, 13
Alveolar dead space, 15
Alveolar hypoventilation
    acute respiratory failure and,
        138-139
    pulmonary hypertension and,
        108
Alveolar oxygen tension, 13
Alveolar septa, 70
Alveoli, 5-8
    adult respiratory distress
        syndrome and, 142-143
    chest configuration inspection,
        35-36
    chronic obstructive pulmonary
        disease and, 71-72
    distribution of ventilation and, 11
    elastance and, 10
    oxygenation and, 16
    primary lobule and, 6
    rales and, 48
    ventilation control and, 19
    ventilation-perfusion
        mismatching, 16
Alveolitis (allergic), 91, 94-95
Aminophylline, 77
Ammonia, 98-99
Ampicillin, 78
Anatomic dead space, 15
Anemia, 36
Anemic hypoxia, 18
Angiography
    pulmonary embolism, 106
    pulmonary hypertension, 110
Angle of Louis, 4
Ankle edema, 76. See also
    Pulmonary edema

Antibiotic therapy. See also
        Pharmacology
    acute respiratory failure, 141
    chronic obstructive pulmonary
        disease, 78
    empyema, 119
    hemothorax, 133
    lung abscess, 115
Anticoagulants, 106
Anxiety
    chronic obstructive pulmonary
        disease, 78-79
    neuromuscular disease, 86
    pulmonary embolism, 105
Aorta, 8
Aortic arch, 19
Aortic bodies, 19
Aortic tear, 131
Apnea
    central nervous system
        depression, 86
    inspection, 38
Apneustic center, 19
ARDS. See Adult respiratory
        distress syndrome
ARF. See Acute respiratory failure
Arsenic exposure, 127
Arterial blood and blood gases
    acid-base balance, 58-64
    acute respiratory failure, 139
    adult respiratory distress
        syndrome, 144-145
    blood sample drawing, 58
    chemoreceptors and, 19
    chronic obstructive pulmonary
        disease, 75
    hydrogen ion concentration, 18
    hypoxemia, 18
    interpretation of, 58-64
Arterial oxygen tension, 13
Arytenoid cartilages, 3-4
Asbestos exposure
    occupational lung disease, 90-91
    pulmonary tumors and, 127
Asbestosis, 92-93
Aspiration
    adult respiratory distress

syndrome and, 143
lung abscess and, 120
right bronchus, 4
Assist/control ventilation, 182
Asterixis, 74
Asthma
  assessment, 52-53
  auscultation, 49
  chronic obstructive pulmonary
    disease and, 71
  lamina propria, 4
  occupational, 90-91, 94-95
  patient history, 26
  smoking and, 73
  work of breathing and, 11
Atelectasis
  adult respiratory distress
    syndrome and, 142-143, 146
  assessment, 50-51, 86
  auscultation, 48
  diffuse, 84
  hypoxemia and, 18
  palpation, 41
  percussion, 43
  restrictive lung disease and, 84
  segmental, 84
  surfactant and, 7, 10
Auscultation, 43-51
  abnormal breath sounds, 48
  adult respiratory distress
    syndrome, 144
  adventitious breath sounds, 48-49
  atelectasis, 86
  central nervous system
    depression, 86
  children, 46
  normal breath sounds, 46-48
  palpation and, 41
  postoperative patients, 87
  pulmonary edema, 107
  pulmonary embolism, 105
  stethoscope, 43
  technique, 44-45
  voice sounds, 50-51

B

Bagging. See Manual ventilation
  (bagging)

Baroreceptors, 19
Barrel chest, 35
Bedridden patients, 35
Bellows mechanism, impaired, 18
Benign bronchial adenoma, 126
Benign lung tumor, 126
Bicarbonate ion, 58-59, 62
Bilateral chest expansion, 41
Bischloromethyl ether exposure,
  127
Black lung disease (coal workers'
  pneumoconiosis), 92-93
Blood
  pulmonary embolism and, 104
  sputum and, 26
Blood flow
  adult respiratory distress
    syndrome, 142
  perfusion and, 13
Blood gases. See Arterial blood
  and blood gases
Blood oxygen transport, 17-18
Blood pressure, 107
Body size, 34
Body temperature
  atelectasis, 86
  blood oxygen transport and, 18
  infection and, 78
  postoperative patients, 87
  pulmonary embolism, 105
  skin inspection, 35
  tuberculosis, 120-121
Bone, 126
Brachial plexus, injury, 131
Bradypnea, 86
Brain
  respiration regulation and, 19, 76
  restrictive lung disease and, 84
  tumor metastasis to, 126
Breath sounds, 44, 46-48
Breathing. See Expiration;
    Inspiration; Ventilation
Breathing dysfunction, 8
Breathing patterns, 38
Briggs adapter, 167
Bronchi. See Bronchus
Bronchial adenoma (benign), 126

Bronchial circulation, 8-9
Bronchial epithelium, 126
Bronchial hygiene, 77-78
Bronchiectasis, 49
Bronchiolar collapse, 70
Bronchioles
    adult respiratory distress
        syndrome, 142
    anatomy, 5
    arteriole/venule and, 8
    asthma and, 70
Bronchitis, 70
    asthma and, 71
    auscultation, 49
    chronic obstructive pulmonary
        disease and, 71
    industrial, 90-91, 96-97
Bronchodilator therapy, 77-78
Bronchogenic carcinoma, 126
Bronchophony, 50-51
Bronchopleural fistula, 115
Bronchoscopy, 87
Bronchospasm, 70
Bronchus
    anatomy, 5
    fracture, 134-135
    lung abscess and, 115
    mainstem, 4-5
    squamous cell carcinoma, 126
Brown lung (byssinosis), 91, 94-95
Bullet wounds, 130
Burns, 138
Byssinosis (brown lung), 91, 94-95

C

Cachectic patient, 34
Cancer. *See also* Pulmonary
        tumors
    lung abscess and, 120
    occupational lung disease,
        90-91, 96-97
    pulmonary hypertension and,
        108
    pulmonary tumors, 126-127
    See also Pulmonary tumors
Capillaries, 142-143
    damage to, 106
Carbon dioxide, 13

narcosis, 76-77
retention, 72
Carbon monoxide poisoning, 18-19
Carbonic acid, 58-59
Cardiac catheterization, 110
Cardiac output
    adult respiratory distress
        syndrome and, 146
    blood oxygen transport and, 17
    chronic obstructive pulmonary
        disease and, 75
    hypoxemia and, 18
    hypoxia and, 18
Cardiac tamponade, 133-134
Cardiopulmonary resuscitation
        (CPR)
    chest trauma, 130
    manual ventilation and, 176
Carina, 4
Carotid arteries, 19
Carotid bodies, 19
Cartilage, 4
Central nervous system
        depression
    assessment of, 86
    restrictive lung disease and, 84
Cerebrospinal fluid, 19
Cervical spine fracture, 8
Chemoreceptors
    brain, 76
    peripheral, 18-19
    ventilation control, 19
Chemotherapy, 127
Chest. *See also* Thorax
    configuration, 35-36
    expansion, 40-41
    vibration, 173
Chest pain
    patient history and, 25
    pulmonary embolism and, 105
    pulmonary tumor, 127
Chest physiotherapy (CPT), 170-174
    chronic obstructive pulmonary
        disease and, 78
    contusion of lung, 133
    hazards of, 173
    indications for, 173

lung abscess, 115
types of, 171-173
Chest trauma, 130-135
See also Trauma
acute respiratory failure and, 138
cardiac tamponade, 133-134
classification, 130-131
contusion of lung, 133
diaphragmatic injuries, 134
flail chest, 131-132
fracture of trachea/bronchus,
134-135
hemothorax, 133
pneumothorax, 132
rib fracture, 131
Cheyne-Stokes respiration, 38
Chlorine, 98-99
Chromate exposure, 127
Chronic conditions, 24, 26
Chronic obstructive pulmonary
disease (COPD), 70-79
acute respiratory failure and,
76, 138-139
arterial blood gases and, 75
asthma and, 70-71
auscultation, 48-49
chronic bronchitis and, 70
clubbing and, 40
CO_2 narcosis and, 76-77
complications of, 75-77
cor pulmonale and, 75-76
emphysema and, 70
etiology, 72-73
incidence, 70
lab studies, 75
nursing diagnosis, 79
occupational lung diasease
and, 91
pathophysiology, 71-72
pneumonia and, 76
pulmonary function studies, 74
pulmonary hypertension and,
108
radiology, 74
signs and symptoms, 73-74
treatment, 77-79
ulcers and, 77

work of breathing and, 11
Cigarette and cigar smoking. *See*
Tobacco smoking
Cilia and ciliated epithelium, 2, 4
chronic bronchitis and, 70
function, 6
mucus and, 40
Clubbing (of fingers)
chronic obstructive pulmonary
disease and, 74
inspection, 40
Coal workers' pneumoconiosis
(black lung disease), 92-93
Collagen disease, 108
Comatose patients, 49
Compliance (lung), 10
adult respiratory distress
syndrome, 146
restrictive lung disease, 84
work of breathing and, 11
Congestive heart failure, 44
Continuous positive airway
pressure (CPAP), 183
Contraceptives, oral, 105
Controlled mechanical
ventilation, 182
Contusion of the lung, 133
COPD. *See* Chronic obstructive
pulmonary disease (COPD)
Coping mechanisms, 27
Cor pulmonale (right heart failure)
chronic obstructive pulmonary
disease, 70-72, 74-76
occupational lung disease and,
100
pulmonary hypertension,109-110
Corticosteroids, 146-147
Cough and coughing
abdominal muscles and, 8
chronic bronchitis and, 70
chronic obstructive pulmonary
disease, 74
infection and, 78
inspection, 37-40
patient history and, 25-26
postoperative, 87
pulmonary embolism and, 105

pulmonary tumor and, 127
Cough reflex, 6, 38-39
Coughing technique, 175
Coughing therapy, 87
CPAP. *See* Continuous positive
  airway pressure (CPAP)
CPT. *See* Chest physiotherapy
  (CPT)
Cricoid cartilage, 2-3
Cyanide poisoning, 18-19
Cyanosis
  adult respiratory distress
    syndrome, 144
  chronic obstructive pulmonary
    disease, 74
  pulmonary edema, 107
  pulmonary embolism, 105
  skin color inspection, 36

D
Dead space, 15
Death. *See* Mortality rates
Deep breathing, 174-175
  surfactant and, 7
Diaphoresis
  adult respiratory distress
    syndrome, 144
  chronic obstructive pulmonary
    disease, 74
  skin inspection, 35
Diaphragm
  anatomy of, 7-8
  auscultation, 48
  chronic obstructive pulmonary
    disease, 74
  inspection and, 37
  paralyzed, 48
Diaphragmatic breathing, 174
Diaphragmatic injuries, 134
Diet, 90
Diffusion, 14
  hypoxemia and, 18
  lung and, 11, 13
Digitalis, 107
Diplococcus pneumoniae, 75,
  76, 78, 114
Disease states
  accessory muscle respiration

and, 8
auscultation, 47
diffusion and, 13
noncompliant lung and, 10
oxygenation and, 16
pulmonary function tests
  and, 13
ventilation/perfusion
  relationship, 14-16
work of breathing and, 11
Diuretics, 107
Drug overdose
  acute respiratory failure
    and, 138
  adult respiratory distress
    syndrome and, 143
  intermittent positive pressure
    breathing therapy, 168
Drugs. *See* Pharmacology
Dust. *See* Irritants
Dyspnea
  atelectasis, 86
  on exertion (DOE), 38
  inspection, 37, 38
  neuromuscular disease, 86
  patient history, 25
  pulmonary edema, 107
  pulmonary embolism, 105
  pulmonary fibrosis, 87

E
Edema. *See* Ankle edema;
    Pulmonary edema
Egophony, 51
Elastance, 9-10
Elasticity, 70
Elderly. *See also* Age
  auscultation, 46
  chronic obstructive pulmonary
    disease, 73
  inspection, 35
  oxygen therapy, 168
  pneumonias, 114
  pulmonary embolism, 105
Electric larynx, 160
Electrocardiography, 105
Embolism. *See* Pulmonary

embolism/embolus
Emotion
  mentation inspection, 35
  patient history, 27
Emphysema
  asthma and, 71
  auscultation, 46
  blebs, 41, 43, 48, 70
  chest configuration, 35
  chronic bronchitis and, 70
  chronic obstructive pulmonary
    disease, 71
  elderly, 35
  heredity and, 73
  occupational lung disease and,
    90
  patient history, 26
  stages in severity of, 72
Empyema, 118-120
  lung abscess and, 115
Endotracheal tubes, 151-153
  acute respiratory failure, 141
  assessment, 52-53, 163
  auscultation, 48
  bronchus and, 4
  complications, 153
  cuff management, 157
  extubation, 153
  indications, 151
  intubation, 152
  oxygen therapy and, 167
  tracheostomy tubes compared,
    156-157
Environmental factors. *See also*
    Occupational lung disease
  cancer, 90
  patient history, 26-27
Enzymes, 73
Eosinophilia, 75
Epidemiology
  chronic obstructive pulmonary
    disease, 70
  occupational lung disease, 90
  pneumonias, 114
  pulmonary tumors, 126-127
Epidermoid (squamous cell)
    carcinoma, 126

Epiglottis, 2
Epinephrine, 77
Epithelium, 4,6
Esophagus, 4
Ethambutol, 121
Eupnea, 38
Exercise
  patient history, 25
  pulmonary embolism, 106
  ventilation control, 19
Expectorants, 78
Expectoration, 70
Expiration. *See also* Inspiration;
    Ventilation
  abdominal muscles, 8
  active, increased, 11
  forced vital capacity, 11
  intercostal muscles, 8
  lung-thorax relationship, 9
  neurocontrol of, 19
Expiratory air flow obstruction, 70
Expiratory reserve volume (ERV),
    12, 84

F

Face tents (oxygen therapy), 167
Family
  chronic obstructive pulmonary
    disease, 79
  patient history, 26-27
  pulmonary tumor, 127
Flail chest, 131-132
  inspection, 37
Flow-volume curves, 11
Fluids
  adult respiratory distress
    syndrome, 143, 145-146
  chronic obstructive pulmonary
    disease, 78
Forced expiratory volume (FEV), 13
  chronic obstructive pulmonary
    disease, 74
  lung volumes, 11
Foreign matter
  cilia/mucus and, 6
  coughing, 38
  larynx, 2
  macrophages, 7

Fractures. *See also* Rib fracture
  pulmonary embolism and, 105
  sternum, 37, 131
  trachea/bronchus, 134-135
Fremitus
  atelectasis, 86
  palpation, 41
  pulmonary fibrosis, 87
Functional residual capacity
  (FRC), 13
  adult respiratory distress
    syndrome, 146
  chronic obstructive pulmonary
    disease, 74
Funnel chest (pectus excavatum), 36

G

Gas exchange
  adult respiratory distress
    syndrome, 146
  alveoli and, 6
  chronic obstructive pulmonary
    disease, 72
  diffusion and, 11, 13
  lung parenchyma, 5
  oxygenation and, 16
  pulmonary edema, 107
  ventilation/perfusion
    relationship, 14-16
Glottis, 2
Goblet cells, 6
Gram-negative aerobic bacilli, 114
Guillain-Barré syndrome
  acute respiratory failure and,
    138
  restrictive lung disease and, 85

H

Haemophilus influenzae, 75-76, 78
Harsh vesicular breath sounds, 46
Headache
  chronic obstructive pulmonary
    disease, 74
  mentation, inspection, 35
Heart. *See also entries under*
    Cardiac; Cardio-
  blood oxygen transport and, 17
  chest pain and, 25

  chronic obstructive pulmonary
    disease and, 72, 74
  oxygen therapy, 168
  percussion, 43
  perfusion, 13
  pulmonary circulation, 8
  pulmonary embolism, 104-105
Heart disease
  clubbing, 40
  occupational lung disease, 91
  pulmonary hypertension, 108
Heart failure. *See also* Cor
    pulmonale (right heart failure)
  left, 106
Hematologic disorders, 143
Hemoglobin
  acid-base balance, 59
  blood oxygen transport, 17-18
  hypoxia and, 18
Hemoglobin-oxygen affinity, 18
Hemoptysis
  benign bronchial adenoma, 126
  pulmonary embolism, 105
  pulmonary tumor, 127
Hemothorax, 130, 133
Henderson-Hasselbalch equation,
    59
Heparin, 106
Heredity, 73
Hering-Breuer reflex, 19
Hernia, 26
Hilus, 7
Hirsute patients, 44
History. *See* Patient history
Hobbies, 26
Humidification
  chronic obstructive pulmonary
    disease, 77-78
  oxygen therapy, 167
Hydration, 35
Hydrogen ion
  acid-base balance, 58, 62
  blood oxygen transport, 18
  lungs and, 59
Hypercapnia
  acute respiratory failure and,
    138-140

adult respiratory distress
syndrome and, 142
chronic obstructive pulmonary
disease and, 72, 75-76
mentation, inspection, 35
Hypercoagulability, 104
Hypersensitivity diseases, 91, 94-97
Hypertension. *See* Blood
pressure; Pulmonary
hypertension
Hyperventilation
adult respiratory distress
syndrome, 143, 146
inspection, 38
respiratory alkalosis, 62
Hypocapnia, 143-144
Hypoperfusion, 142
Hypoventilation
alveolar, primary, 18
inspection, 38
respiratory acidosis, 62
Hypoxemia, 18
acute respiratory failure and, 72
adult respiratory distress
syndrome and, 141-144
chronic obstructive pulmonary
disease and, 72, 75-77
diffusion defects, 13
oxygenation and, 16
pulmonary edema and, 107
pulmonary embolism and, 104
pulmonary hypertension and,
108-110
Hypoxia, 18-19
acute respiratory failure and,
139-140
central nervous system
depression, 86
chronic obstructive pulmonary
disease, 76
cyanosis and, 36
mentation inspection, 35
oxygenation and, 16
postsurgical, 85
pulmonary edema, 107
pulmonary hypertension and,
108

Hypoxic hypoxia, 18

I

Immobility, 105
Immune system, 108
Immunotherapy, 127
Incentive spirometry, 170-171
pulmonary embolism, 106
restrictive lung disease, 87
surfactant and, 7
Industrial accidents, 130
Industrial bronchitis, 91, 96-97.
See also Occupational lung
disease
Infancy
cricoid cartilage, 3
inspection, 34-35
Infection. *See also* Lung
infections
acute respiratory failure and,
138, 141
adult respiratory distress
syndrome, 143
chronic bronchitis and, 70
chronic obstructive pulmonary
disease and, 73, 75, 76, 78
inspection and, 37, 40
lung abscess and, 120
occupational lung disease and,
100
patient history and, 26
pulmonary fibrosis and, 86
Influenza, 114
Innervation
abdominal muscles, 8
bronchi, 5
diaphragm, 8
intercostal muscles, 8
lamina propria, 4
lung parenchyma, 25
pleura, 7
Inspection, 34-40
age level and, 34-35
body size and, 34
characteristics of respirations,
37
chest configuration, 35-36

clubbing, 40
cough and secretions, 37-40
mentation, 35
posture, 35
skin color, 36
skin quality, 35
vital signs, 40
Inspiration. *See also* Expiration;
Ventilation
accessory muscles and, 8
auscultation, 46
compliance and, 10
diaphragm and, 7
lung-thorax relationship, 9
neurocontrol of, 19
Inspiratory reserve volume (IRV),
12, 84
Intensive care units, 140, 145
Intercostal muscles
anatomy, 8
inspection, 37
posture inspection, 35
Intercostal space, 43
Intermittent mandatory
ventilation, 182
Intermittent positive pressure
breathing (IPPB) therapy,
168-169
acute respiratory failure, 141
controversy in, 168
hazards in, 169
incentive spirometry
contrasted, 171
indications for, 168-169
surfactant and, 7
Interstitial disease, 108
Interstitial elastic fibers, 10
Intrapulmonary shunting, 18
Intubation. *See also* Airway
management
bronchus and, 4
infants and, 3
positive pressure mechanical
ventilators, 180
trachea and, 4
IPPB therapy. *See* Intermittent
positive pressure breathing

(IPPB) therapy
Irritants
occupational disorders, 91,
96-99
pulmonary fibrosis and, 86
Isoetharine, 77
Isoniazid, 121
Isoproterenol hydrochloride, 77

J
Joints, proprioceptors, 19

K
Kidney
acid-base balance and, 62
chronic obstructive pulmonary
disease, 75
Knife wounds, 130
Kyphoscoliosis
patient history, 26
pulmonary hypertension and,
108
Kyphosis, 36

L
Laboratory tests
chronic obstructive pulmonary
disease, 75
percussion and, 43
pulmonary embolism, 105
Lactic acidemia, 18
Lamina propria (submucosa), 4
Large-cell carcinoma, 126
Laryngopharynx, 2
Larynx (voice box), 2-4
Left bronchus, 4-5
Liver
chronic obstructive pulmonary
disease and, 74, 76
clubbing and, 40
diaphragmatic injuries and, 134
metastasis to, 126
Lobar atelectasis, 84. *See
also* Atelectasis
Lobar bronchi, 5
Lobectomy, 115
Lobule, primary, 6
Localized fibrosis, 85-87

Lower airway, 2, 4-5
Lung
  acid-base balance and, 59, 62
  auscultation, 44
  blood supply, 9
  bronchi and, 5
  chronic obstructive pulmonary
    disease and, 72
  diffusion and, 11, 13-14
  hypoxemia and, 18
  metastasis to, 126
  neurocontrol of ventilation, 19
  occupational history and, 26-27
  oxygenation and oxygen
    transport, 16-19
  perfusion and, 13
  physiology, 9-19
  posture inspection and, 35
  thorax and, 7, 9
  ventilation/perfusion
    relationship, 14-16
Lung abscess, 115, 118
  causes, 115, 120
  nursing goals, 115, 118
  palpation, 41
  treatment, 115
Lung cancer. See Cancer;
    Pulmonary tumors
Lung collapse, 132
Lung infections. See also Infection
  classification, 114
  empyema, 118-120
  lung abscess, 115, 118
  pneumonias, 114-115
  tuberculosis, 120-122
Lung mass, 41
Lung parenchyma
  anatomy of, 5-6
  auscultation, 47
  bronchial breath sounds, 48
  pain and, 25
Lung tumors. See Cancer;
    Pulmonary tumors
Lung volumes, 11-13. See also
    entries under names of lung
    volumes
Lymphatic supply and system

  alveolar cells and, 6
  bronchi, 5
  lamina propria, 4
  mucus absorption and, 40
Lymphoid tissue, 2

M

Macrophages
  alveolar fluid lining, 7
  mucus and, 40
Mainstem bronchi, 4-5
Manual ventilation (bagging),
    175-177
Manubrium, 4
Masks (oxygen therapy), 166-167
Maximum midexpiratory flow
    rate (MMEFR)
  chronic obstructive pulmonary
    disease and, 74
  lung volumes, 11, 13
Maximum voluntary ventilation
    (MVV), 11, 13
Mechanical ventilation, 180-184
  adult respiratory distress
    syndrome and, 146
  assessment, 184
  classification of ventilators,
    180-181
  contusion of lung, 133
  flail chest, 132
  indications, 180-181
  problems with, 183
  restrictive lung disease, 85, 87
  volume ventilator functions
    and settings, 181-183
Mediastinum, 126
Medulla (brain), 19
Mentation, 35
Metabolic acidosis, 60-62
  compensation for, 63
  medical correction of, 64
Metabolic alkalosis, 60-62
  compensation for, 63
  medical correction of, 64
Metabolic disorders, 143
Metabolism
  anaerobic, 18

hypoxia and, 18
skin inspection, 35
ventilation and, 19
Metaproterenol, 77
Metastases
pulmonary hypertension and, 108
pulmonary tumors and, 126
Methylxanthines, 76-77
Minute ventilation (V_E), 11
Mixed dust pneumoconioses, 92-93
Mortality rates
bronchogenic carcinoma, 126
chronic obstructive pulmonary disease, 70
occupational lung disease, 90
pneumonias, 114
pulmonary hypertension, 109
pulmonary tumors, 126-127
Mouth, 2
Mucous glands, 4
Mucus
anatomy and, 6
asthma, chronic bronchitis and, 70
chronic obstructive pulmonary disease and, 76
content of, 6
coughing and, 40
terminal bronchioles and, 5
Muscle proprioceptors, 19
Muscles of ventilation
anatomy, 7-8
inspection, 37
neuromuscular disease, 85
work of breathing, 11
Muscular dystrophy
acute respiratory failure and, 138
restrictive lung disease and, 85
Myasthenia gravis
acute respiratory failure and, 138
hypoxemia and, 18
restrictive lung disease and, 85
Mycobacterium tuberculosis, 120
Mycoplasma, 114

N

Nares, 2
Nasal endotracheal tubes, 152. *See also* Endotracheal tubes
Nasal septum, 2
Nasopharyngeal airway, 150-151, 162.*See also* Airway management
Nasopharynx, 2
Nebulizers (oxygen therapy), 167
Neck injury, 131
Neck vein distention, 76
Negative pressure mechanical ventilators, 180
Neonates. *See* Infancy
Neoplasm, 43
Nerves. *See* Innervation
Neurology
chronic obstructive pulmonary disease, 74
oxygen therapy, 168
Neuromuscular disease
acute respiratory failure and, 138
assessment of, 86
restrictive lung disease and, 85
Nitrogen dioxide exposure, 98-99
Noncompliant lung, 10. *See also* Compliance (lung)
Nose, 2
Nosocomial pneumonia, 114 116-119

O

Obesity
acute respiratory failure and, 138
auscultation and, 46
inspection and, 34
pulmonary embolism and, 105
pulmonary hypertension and, 108
Obstructive disease. *See also* Chronic obstructive pulmonary disease (COPD)
pulmonary function tests, 13
Occupational history. *See also* Patient history

lung disease and, 91, 100
patient history and, 26-27
Occupational lung disease, 90-100
asthma, 94-95
cancer, 96-97
chronic obstructive pulmonary
disease, 73
diagnosis, 90-91
incidence, 90
major types, 91-99
nursing goals, 100
pulmonary tumors, 127
Oral endotracheal tubes, 152.
See also Endotracheal tubes
Oropharyngeal airway, 150, 162
Oropharynx, 2
Orthopnea
inspection, 38
patient history, 25
Oxtriphylline, 77
Oxygen concentration, 182
Oxygen diffusibility, 13
Oxygen therapy
acute respiratory failure, 141
adult respiratory distress
syndrome, 144-145
chronic obstructive pulmonary
disease, 76-77
humidification and, 78
hypoxemia and, 16, 18
manual ventilation and, 176-177
pulmonary edema, 107
pulmonary embolism, 106
pulmonary hypertension, 110
restrictive lung disease, 85
techniques, 166-168
Oxygen transport, 17-18
Oxygenation
lung and, 16
skin color inspection, 36
Oxyhemoglobin dissociation
curve, 17-18
Ozone, 98-99

P

Pain. *See* Chest pain
Palpation, 40-41
Papilledema, 74

Paradoxical chest movement, 131
Parietal pleura, 7
Paroxysmal nocturnal dyspnea
(PND), 38
Patchy atelectasis, 84
Patient education
adult respiratory distress
syndrome, 147
chronic obstructive pulmonary
disease, 78-79
occupational lung disease, 100
pneumonia, 115
pulmonary embolism, 106
pulmonary tumors, 127
Patient history, 24-30
acute vs. chronic condition, 24
chest trauma, 130
chief complaint, 24
contributing factors and, 26-27
inspection and, 38
occupational disorders, 91,
92-100
onset of illness, 25
psychosocial/emotional
factors, 27
rationale for, 24
sample questionnaire, 27-30
symptoms and, 25-26
Pectoralis muscle, 8
Pectus carinatum (pigeon breast),
36
Pectus excavatum (funnel chest), 36
PEEP. *See* Positive end expiratory
pressure (PEEP)
Peptic ulcer disease, 77
Percussion
assessment, 42-43
atelectasis, 86
chest physiotherapy, 172-173
chronic obstructive pulmonary
disease, 74
pulmonary fibrosis, 87
Perfusion, 14-16
Perfusion lung scan, 105
Pericardial aspiration, 134
Pericardiotomy, 134
Peripheral cyanosis, 36.

See also Cyanosis
Personality change, 35
pH. *See* Acid-base balance
    disturbances; Hydrogen ion
Phagocytic cells, 7
Pharmacology
  acute respiratory failure, 141
  adult respiratory distress
    syndrome, 145-147
  chronic obstructive pulmonary
    disease, 76-78
  empyema, 119
  hand-held aerosol/mini-
    nebulizer therapy, 169
  hemothorax, 133
  intermittent positive pressure
    breathing therapy, 169
  lung abscess, 115
  oxygen therapy, 166
  pneumonias, 114, 117, 119
  pulmonary edema, 107
  pulmonary embolism, 106
  tuberculosis, 121
Pharynx (throat), 2
Phosgene, 98-99
Phosphates, 59
Phospholipid, 7
Phrenic nerve, 8
Pigeon breast (pectus
    carinatum), 36
Pipe smoking. *See* Tobacco
    smoking
Pleura
  anatomy, 7
  palpation, 41
Pleural cavity, 7
Pleural effusion
  auscultation, 48
  palpation, 41
  percussion, 43
Pleural fluid, 84
Pleural pressure, 9
Pneumoconioses, 91-93
Pneumocytes, 142
Pneumonia(s), 114-115
  acute respiratory failure
    and, 138

assessment, 50-51
  atelectasis and, 84
  auscultation, 48-49
  chronic obstructive pulmonary
    disease and, 70,76
  classification/etiology, 114
  contusion of lung and, 133
  hypostatic, 84
  incidence, 114
  lung abscess and, 115
  nosocomial, 114, 116-119
  nursing goals in, 114-115
  palpation, 41
  patient history and, 26
  pulmonary hypertension and,
    108
Pneumonitis, 86
Pneumotaxic center, 19
Pneumothorax, 132
  adult respiratory distress
    syndrome and, 146
  assessment, 52-53
  atelectasis, 84
  auscultation, 48
  chest trauma, 130
  palpation, 41
  percussion, 43
  rib fracture, 131
  tension pneumothorax, 132
  treatment, 132
Poliomyelitis
  acute respiratory failure and,
    138
  restrictive lung disease and,
    85
Pollutants. *See* Air pollution
Polycythemia
  chronic obstructive pulmonary
    disease, 75
  cyanosis and, 36
Pons, 19
Pores of Kohn, 11
Position. *See* Postural drainage;
    Posture
Positive end expiratory pressure
    (PEEP)
  adult respiratory distress

syndrome, 146
mechanical ventilators, 183
Positive pressure mechanical
    ventilators, 180-181
Postoperative patients. *See also*
    Surgery
  acute respiratory failure, 138
  assessment, 87
  auscultation, 49
  empyema, 118
  incentive spirometry, 171
  pulmonary embolism and,
    104-105
  restrictive lung disease and,
    84-85
Postural drainage
  bronchi and, 5
  chest physiotherapy, 171-172
  chronic obstructive pulmonary
    disease, 78
  contusion of lung, 133
  restrictive lung disease, 87
Posture
  auscultation and, 44
  inspection and, 35
Pregnancy, 105
Premature infants, 34-35
Pressure-cycled ventilators,
    180-181
Pressure setting (respirators), 182
Proprioceptors, 19
Protein, 59
Psychosocial factors, 27
Pulmonary abscess, 86
Pulmonary angiography
  pulmonary embolism, 106
  pulmonary hypertension, 110
Pulmonary artery thermodilution
    catheter, 13
Pulmonary artery wedge pressure
    (PAWP), 145
Pulmonary circulation, 8
Pulmonary consolidation, 86
Pulmonary edema, 106-107
  assessment, 52-53, 107
  auscultation, 48-49
  causes, 106

noncompliant lung and, 10
nursing goals, 107
treatment, 107
work of breathing and, 11
Pulmonary embolism/embolus,
    104-106
  auscultation, 49
  etiology, 104
  hypoxemia and, 18
  lung abscess and, 115, 120
  nursing goals, 106
  pulmonary hypertension and,
    108
  treatment, 106
  ventilation/perfusion
    relationship, 15
Pulmonary fibrosis, 10
  assessment of, 87
  generalized, 86-87
  hypoxemia and, 18
  interstitial, 48
  restrictive lung disease and,
    85-86
Pulmonary function studies
  chronic obstructive pulmonary
    disease, 74
  pulmonary hypertension, 110
  significance, 13
Pulmonary hypertension, 109-110
  causes, 108
  nursing goals, 110
  treatment, 110
Pulmonary rehabilitation
    program, 79
Pulmonary tumors, 126-127. *See
    also* Cancer
  auscultation, 48
  classification, 126
  incidence and etiology, 126-127
  lung abscess and, 115
  nursing goals, 127
  pulmonary embolism and, 105
  treatment, 127
Pulmonary vascular disease,
    104-110
  chronic obstructive pulmonary
    disease, 71

pulmonary edema, 106-107
pulmonary embolism, 104-106
pulmonary hypertension,
    107-110
Pulmonary vascular resistance,
    108-109
Pulmonary vessels, 7
Pursed lip breathing, 174-175
    chronic obstructive pulmonary
        disease, 74
    inspection and, 37

R

Radiation therapy, 127
Radiology
    adult respiratory distress
        syndrome, 144
    atelectasis, 84
    chronic obstructive pulmonary
        disease, 74
    diaphragmatic injury, 134
    empyema, 120
    endotracheal tube placement,
        152
    lung tumors, 126
    percussion, 43
    pulmonary embolism, 105-106
    pulmonary tumors, 127
    tuberculosis, 121
Rales. See also Auscultation
    auscultation, 48
    false, 44
    rhonchi, 48
Receptor responses, 19
Red blood cells
    chronic obstructive pulmonary
        disease, 75
    pulmonary circulation, 8
Residual volume (RV), 84
Respiration. See Expiration;
    Inspiration; Ventilation
Respiratory acidosis, 60-62
    acid-base balance, 58
    chronic obstructive pulmonary
        disease, 75
    compensation for, 63
    medical correction of, 63-64
Respiratory alkalosis, 60-62

acid-base balance, 58
    compensation for, 63
    medical correction of, 64
Respiratory distress syndrome.
    See also Adult respiratory
    distress syndrome (ARDS)
Respiratory rate
    mechanical ventilation, 181
    oxygenation and, 16
Respiratory therapy, 166-177
    atelectasis, 84
    chest physiotherapy, 170-174
    deep breathing, 174-175
    hand-held aerosol/mini-
        nebulizer therapy, 169-170
    incentive spirometry, 170-171
    intermittent positive pressure
        breathing therapy, 168-169
    manual ventilation, 175-177
    oxygen therapy, 166-168
Restrictive lung disease, 84-87
    adult respiratory distress
        syndrome, 84, 86
    atelectasis, 84
    central nervous system
        depression, 84
    neuromuscular disease, 85
    nursing goals, 87
    postoperative, 84-85
    pulmonary consolidation, 85
    pulmonary fibrosis, 85-86
    pulmonary function tests and,
        13
    treatment, 87
    types, 84-86
Rhonchi, 41, 48-49
Rib fracture
    chest trauma, 131
    coughing, 38
    flail chest and, 131
    inspection, 37
    patient history and, 26
    trachea/bronchus fracture and,
        134
    treatment, 131
Ribs, 8
Rifampin, 121

S

Sample patient questionnaire, 27-30
Sarcoidosis, 108
Scalene muscle, 8
Scars, 36
Scleroderma, 108
Scoliosis, 36
Secretions
  auscultation, 48
  coughing and, 40
  inspection, 37-40
  retained, 84
Segmental breathing, 175
Segmental bronchi, 5
Serous gland, 4
Sex differences
  chronic obstructive pulmonary disease, 70
  pulmonary hypertension, 107-108
  pulmonary tumors, 126
Shock
  adult respiratory distress syndrome and, 142-143
  hypoxemia and, 18
  pulmonary embolism and, 105
Shock lung. See Adult respiratory distress syndrome (ARDS)
Shortness of breath
  chronic obstructive pulmonary disease and, 74
  infection and, 78
  inspection, 37
  patient history, 27
Sighs (mechanical ventilation), 183
Silent gap, 47
Silicosis, 92-93
Skin color, 36
Skin quality, 35
Sleep, 74
Small-cell anaplastic carcinoma, 126
Smell, 2
Smog, 73. See also Air pollution
Smoking. See Tobacco smoking
Snoring, 38

Soft palate, 2
Speech, 2
Spinal cord injury, 85
Sputum
  chronic obstructive pulmonary disease and, 74
  content of, 6
  infection and, 78
  patient history and, 25-26
Sputum culture
  antibiotic therapy and, 78
  chronic obstructive pulmonary disease and, 75
  tuberculosis and, 121
Squamous cell (epidermoid) carcinoma, 126
Stagnant hypoxia, 18
Staphylococcus aureus, 114
Sternocleidomastoid muscles, 8, 37
Sternum, 4
Steroids, 77-78
Stertorous breathing, 38
Stethoscope, 43
Streptokinase, 106
Streptomycin, 121
Stress, 90
Stressors, 27
Stridor, 38
Submucosal glands, 6
Suctioning
  chronic obstructive pulmonary disease, 78
  endotracheal tubes, 152
  nasopharyngeal airway, 150-151
  restrictive lung disease, 87
  right bronchus, 4
  tracheostomy tubes, 158, 160-161
Sulphur dioxide exposure, 96-97
Support systems, 27
Surfactant
  adult respiratory distress syndrome, 142-143
  alveolar fluid lining, 7
  alveoli and, 6
  mechanical ventilation, 183
Surgery. See also Postoperative patients

cardiac tamponade, 134
diaphragmatic injuries, 134
lung abscess, 115
pulmonary embolism, 106
pulmonary tumors, 127
tracheostomy, 154
Swan-Ganz catheter, 145
Sympathomimetics, 76-77
Synchronized intermittent
mandatory ventilation, 183
Syncope, 105

T

Tachycardia
adult respiratory distress
syndrome, 144
chronic obstructive pulmonary
disease, 74
pulmonary edema, 107
pulmonary embolism, 105
Tachypnea
chronic obstructive pulmonary
disease, 74
inspection, 38
pulmonary embolism, 105
Tactile fremitus, 41. See also
Fremitus
Tension pneumothorax, 132. See
also Pneumothorax
Terbutaline, 77
Terminal bronchioles, 5
Tetanus, 85
Tetracycline, 78
Theophylline, 77
Thickened pleura, 41
Thoracic cage, 7
Thoracic injury. See Chest trauma
Thoracic lesions, 84
Thoracic surgery, 85
Thoracocentesis, 119, 133
Thoracotomy, 134
Thorax
anatomy, 7
lung-thorax relationship, 9
obesity and, 34
Throat, 2
Thrombosis, deep vein, 104-105

Thyroid cartilage, 2, 4
Tidal volume
mechanical ventilation, 181
restrictive lung disease, 84
Time-cycled ventilators, 181
Tissues, 13
Tobacco smoking
cancer and, 90, 127
children, 27
chronic bronchitis and, 70
chronic obstructive pulmonary
disease and, 70, 72-73
coughing and, 38
occupational disorders and, 91,
96-97, 100
patient history, 27
postoperative patients, 85
pulmonary tumors, 90, 127
Tongue, 2, 36
Tonsils, 2
Total lung capacity (TLC), 13
chronic obstructive pulmonary
disease, 74
restrictive lung disease, 84
Toxic hypoxia, 18-19
Toxins. See also Occupational
lung disease
adult respiratory distress
syndrome, 143
patient history, 26-27
pulmonary fibrosis, 86
Trach collars, 167
Trachea (windpipe)
anatomy, 4
bronchi and, 4-5
fracture, 134-135
glottis and, 2
Tracheobronchial hygiene, 141
Tracheobronchial tree
anatomy, 4
chronic bronchitis, 70
lungs and, 7
pulmonary circulation and, 8
submucosal glands, 6
Tracheoesophageal fistula, 4
Tracheostomy and tracheostomy
tubes, 153-162

assessment, 163
characteristics of, 154-156
communication with patient,
    159-161
complications, 154, 156
cuff management, 156-159
endotracheal tubes compared,
    156-157
indications, 153-154
intubation, 154
oxygen therapy and, 167
patient care, 159, 162
positive pressure mechanical
    ventilators, 180
suctioning, 158, 160-161
Trapezius muscle, 8
Trauma. *See also* Chest trauma
    adult respiratory distress
        syndrome, 143
    empyema and, 118
    inspection, 37
    lung abscess and, 115
    pulmonary embolism and, 104-
        105
Tuberculosis, 120-122
    auscultation, 48
    lung abscess and, 115
    nursing goals, 122
    pulmonary fibrosis and, 86
    treatment, 121
Tumors. *See* Cancer; Pulmonary
    tumors
Turbinates (nose), 2

V

Vagus nerve, 19
Vascular obstruction, 108
Vasculitis, 108
Venous admixture, 15
Venous injury, 104
Venous stasis, 104
Ventilation. *See* Expiration;
    Inspiration; Respiration
    defined, 9
    distribution of, 11, 16, 72
    hypoxemia and, 18
    inspection and, 37

lung and, 9-11
lung volumes and, 11-13
muscles and, 7-8
neurocontrol of, 19
work of breathing and, 11
Ventilation lung scan, 105
Ventilation-perfusion
    relationship, 14-16
    chronic obstructive pulmonary
        disease, 72, 76
    contusion of lung, 133
    hypoxemia and, 18
    pulmonary embolism, 104
Ventilators. *See* Mechanical
    ventilation
Ventilatory failure. *See* Acute
    respiratory failure (ARF)
Venturi masks, 166
Vesicular breath sounds, 46
Virchow's triad, 104
Visceral pleura, 7
Vital capacity (VC)
    chronic obstructive pulmonary
        disease, 74
    lung volumes, 11, 13
    postoperative, 85, 87
    restrictive lung disease, 84
Vital signs, 40
Vocal cords
    anatomy, 4
    arytenoid cartilages and, 3
    paralysis, 156
Vocal fremitus, 41. *See also*
    Fremitus
Voice box (larynx), 2-4
Voice sounds, 50-51
Volume-cycled ventilators,
    181-183
Vomitus aspiration, 86, 115, 120

W

Warfarin sodium, 106
Wheezes, 49. *See also*
    Auscultation
    patient history and, 27
    rhonchi and, 48
Whispered pectoriloquy, 51

Windpipe. *See* Trachea
Work of breathing
   chronic obstructive pulmonary
     disease, 71-72
   inspection and, 37
   obesity and, 34
   restrictive lung disease and, 84
   skin inspection and, 35
World Health Organization, 90

X

Xanthines, 77
X-ray. *See* Radiology